O A C L
OXFORD AMERICAN CARDIOLOGY LIBRARY

Interventional Cardiology: Essential Clinician's Guide

This material is not intended to be, and should not be considered, a substitute for medical or other professional advice. Treatment for the conditions described in this material is highly dependent on the individual circumstances. While this material is designed to offer accurate information with respect to the subject matter covered and to be current as of the time it was written, research and knowledge about medical and health issues are constantly evolving, and dose schedules for medications are being revised continually, with new side effects recognized and accounted for regularly. Readers must therefore always check the product information and clinical procedures with the most up-to-date published product information and data sheets provided by the manufacturers and the most recent codes of conduct and safety regulation. Oxford University Press and the authors make no representations or warranties to readers, express or implied, as to the accuracy or completeness of this material, including without limitation that they make no representations or warranties as to the accuracy or efficacy of the drug dosages mentioned in the material. The authors and the publishers do not accept, and expressly disclaim, any responsibility for any liability, loss, or risk that may be claimed or incurred as a consequence of the use and/or application of any of the contents of this material.

The Publisher is responsible for author selection and the Publisher and the Author(s) make all editorial decisions, including decisions regarding content. The Publisher and the Author(s) are not responsible for any product information added to this publication by companies purchasing copies of it for distribution to clinicians.

O A C L
OXFORD AMERICAN CARDIOLOGY LIBRARY

Interventional Cardiology: Essential Clinician's Guide

Debabrata Mukherjee, MD, MS

Chief of Cardiovascular Medicine
Vice Chairman
Department of Internal Medicine
Paul L. Foster School of Medicine
Texas Tech University Health Sciences Center
El Paso, TX

Anthony A. Bavry, MD, MPH

Assistant Professor of Medicine
University of Florida
Gainesville, FL

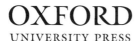
OXFORD
UNIVERSITY PRESS

OXFORD

UNIVERSITY PRESS

Oxford University Press, Inc., publishes works that further
Oxford University's objective of excellence
in research, scholarship, and education.

Oxford New York
Auckland Cape Town Dar es Salaam Hong Kong Karachi
Kuala Lumpur Madrid Melbourne Mexico City Nairobi
New Delhi Shanghai Taipei Toronto

With offices in
Argentina Austria Brazil Chile Czech Republic France Greece
Guatemala Hungary Italy Japan Poland Portugal Singapore
South Korea Switzerland Thailand Turkey Ukraine Vietnam

Published by Oxford University Press, Inc.
198 Madison Avenue, New York, New York 10016
www.oup.com

Oxford is a registered trademark of Oxford University Press

Library of Congress Cataloging-in-Publication Data

Interventional cardiology : essential clinician's guide / [edited by]
Debabrata Mukherjee, Anthony A. Bavry.
p. ; cm. — (Oxford American cardiology library)

Includes bibliographical references and index.

ISBN 978-0-19-973260-9 (regular ed. : alk. paper)—ISBN 978-0-19-539337-8 (standard ed. : alk.
paper)—ISBN 978-0-19-539338-5 (special sale ed. : alk. paper)

1. Heart—Endoscopic surgery—Handbooks, manuals, etc. I. Mukherjee, Debabrata. II. Bavry,
Anthony A. III. Series: Oxford American cardiology library.

[DNLM: 1. Coronary Disease—surgery. 2. Cardiovascular Surgical Procedures—methods.
3. Coronary Disease—therapy.   WG 300 I6442 2010]

RD598.I545 2010

617.4'120597—dc22   2009039473

Contents

Contributors

Khurram Ahmad, MD
Cardiology Fellow
University of Tennessee Health
Sciences Center
Memphis, Tennessee

R. David Anderson, MD
Associate Professor of Medicine
Division of Cardiovascular Medicine
Director, Interventional Cardiology
Director of the Cardiac
Catheterization Laboratory
Shands Hospital
Gainesville, Florida

Saif Anwaruddin, MD
Fellow, Section of Interventional
Cardiology
Heart and Vascular Institute
Cleveland Clinic
Cleveland, Ohio

Amer K. Ardati, MD
University of Michigan
Ann Arbor, Michigan

Rohit Bhatheja, MD
Interventional Fellow,
Division of Cardiovascular Medicine
University of Kentucky
Lexington, Kentucky

Sanjay Bhojraj, MD
Henry Ford Hospital
Detroit, Michigan

Adnan K. Chhatriwalla, MD
Clinical Scholar
Mid America Heart Institute
Saint Luke's Hospital
Kansas City, Missouri

Calvin Choi, MD
Cardiology Fellow
Division of Cardiovascular Medicine
University of Florida
Gainesville, Florida

Pranab Das, MD
Assistant Professor
Division of Cardiology,
Department of Internal
Medicine
University of Tennessee Health
Sciences Center
Memphis, Tennessee

Arijit Dasgupta, MD
Interventional Fellow
Division of Cardiovascular Medicine
University of Kentucky
Lexington, Kentucky

Jose G. Diez, MD
Assistant Professor of Medicine
Director Invasive Cardiology Baylor
Heart Clinic
Director Interventional
Cardiology Research Baylor
College of Medicine
Interventional Cardiology-
Professional Staff
St. Luke's Episcopal Hospital/
Texas Heart Institute
Houston, Texas

Ryan D'Souza, MD
Interventional Fellow
Swiss Cardiovascular Center Bern
University Hospital
Bern, Switzerland

Carl Dragstedt, DO

Fellow in Cardiovascular Medicine
Division of Cardiovascular Medicine
Department of Medicine
University of Florida Health
Science Center
Gainesville, Florida

Hitinder S. Gurm, MBBS

Staff, Interventional Cardiology
Assistant Professor of Medicine
Division of Cardiovascular Medicine
University of Michigan
Cardiovascular Center
Ann Arbor, Michigan

Adam Greenbaum, MD

Associate Director, Cardiac
Catheterization Laboratory
Henry Ford Hospital
Assistant Professor of Medicine
Wayne State University
Detroit, Michigan

Hussam Hamdalla, MD

Gill Heart Institute and Division of
Cardiovascular Medicine
University of Kentucky
Lexington, Kentucky

Thomas J. Helton, DO

Fellow, Interventional Cardiology
Department of Cardiovascular
Medicine
Heart & Vascular Institute
Cleveland Clinic
Cleveland, Ohio

Ion S. Jovin MD, ScD

Assistant Professor of Medicine
Director, Cardiac Catheterization
McGuire Veterans Affairs Medical
Center
Medical College of Virginia
Virginia Commonwealth University
Richmond, Virginia

Sharat Koul, DO

Interventional Fellow
Division of Cardiovascular Medicine
University of Kentucky
Lexington, Kentucky

Dharam J. Kumbhani, MD, SM

Fellow in Cardiovascular Medicine
Cleveland Clinic
Cleveland, Ohio

Michael J. Lim, MD

Interim Director, Division of
Cardiology and
Director, J. Gerard Mudd Cardiac
Catheterization Lab
Associate Professor of Medicine
Saint Louis University
Saint Louis, Missouri

C. Ryan Longnecker, MD

Assistant Professor of Medicine
Division of Cardiology
Saint Louis University Hospital
Saint Louis, Missouri

Bernhard Meier, MD

Professor and Chairman of
Cardiology
Swiss Cardiovascular Center Bern
University Hospital
Bern, Switzerland

Srihari S. Naidu, MD

Director, Cardiac Catheterization
Laboratory
Interventional Cardiology
Fellowship Program and
Hypertrophic Cardiomyopathy
Center
Winthrop University Hospital
Assistant Professor of Medicine
SUNY-Stony Brook School of
Medicine
Mineola, New York

Pritam R. Polkampally, MD

Cardiology Fellow
Division of Cardiology
Medical College of Virginia
Virginia Commonwealth University
Richmond, Virginia

Henri Roukoz, MD, MSc

Division of Cardiology, Department
of Internal Medicine
University of Minnesota Medical
Center
Minneapolis, Minnesota

Mike Sarkees, MD

Internal Medicine Resident
Department of Internal Medicine
Cleveland Clinic
Cleveland, Ohio

Mehdi H. Shishehbor, DO, MPH

Staff, Interventional Cardiology and
Vascular Medicine
Department of Cardiovascular
Medicine
Heart & Vascular Institute, Cleveland
Clinic
Cleveland, Ohio

Inder M. Singh, MD, MS

Fellow, Interventional Cardiology
Division of Cardiovascular Diseases
Mayo Clinic
Rochester, Minnesota

Allyne Topaz, BS

Medical Student
St. George's University School
of Medicine
Grenada

On Topaz, MD

Professor of Medicine and Pathology
Director Interventional Cardiology
McGuire Veterans Affairs Medical
Center
Medical College of Virginia
Virginia Commonwealth University
Richmond, Virginia

James M. Wilson, MD

Director, Cardiology Training
Program
Co-Director, Cardiology Section
Interventional Cardiology-
Professional Staff
St. Luke's Episcopal Hospital/Texas
Heart Institute
Houston, Texas

Khaled M. Ziada, MD

Associate Professor of Medicine
Director, Cardiac Catheterization
Laboratories
Lexington VAMC Director
Cardiovascular Interventional
Fellowship Program
Gill Heart Institute
University of Kentucky
Lexington, Kentucky

Chapter 1

Basic Radiation Principles and Contrast Media

C. Ryan Longnecker and Michael J. Lim

Radiation

Exposure to x-ray radiation is inherent in performing cardiac catheterization or other invasive cardiovascular procedures. Although catheterization techniques have changed vastly over the last 40 years with regards to vascular access, catheters, anticoagulation, and stents, little change has come in the utilization of radiation as the source for imaging. Ultimately, radiation safety in the catheterization lab cannot be emphasized enough, since the long-term effects of radiation may relate directly to significant morbidity and mortality for the operators, staff, and patients.[1] To this end, all hospitals have radiation safety officers and procedures to assure proper education and exposure level monitoring for personnel working in areas utilizing x-ray imaging, as well as for patients undergoing these tests.

There are two major mechanisms whereby radiation harms individuals: deterministic and stochastic. *Deterministic effects* are almost linearly related to the dose received by the subject, and they usually do not occur with radiation exposures below a certain threshold. They are the result of direct toxicity by the x-rays and result from cellular death and biochemical tissue responses. The higher the dose of radiation, the higher the probability a patient will have a more severe deterministic effect. Skin erythema, follicular loss, skin desquamation, bone marrow suppression, sterility, and cataracts are all deterministic effects of radiation exposure.[1,2,3] *Stochastic effects* are random, and can occur with a single x-ray exposure. Stochastic effects result from modification of DNA that can then cause mutation of the cellular structure and tumor formation or heritable genetic defects. The "linear-no-threshold" model of radiation risk is based upon stochastic effects and is used to remind operators that no dose of radiation is safe, but higher doses do pose more risk.[3] Unlike deterministic effects in the skin, stochastic effects can take several years to develop. Radiation-associated leukemia has been seen 2 years after exposure. Solid malignancies generally require about 5 years to develop, but they can occur several decades after exposure. Female breast tissue is a particularly radiosensitive area, and attempts should be made to minimize radiation exposure to that region as much as possible.

Based upon the Biologic Effects of Ionizing Radiation (BEIR) VII report, there was the suggestion that evidence is insufficient to prove that low-dose radiation exposure in the catheterization lab increases an individual's risk of malignancy beyond that from the background radiation he or she receives from living on Earth (approximately 3 mSv/year).[4,5] Although this might be true, it is also clear that both deterministic and stochastic risks are increased with large doses of radiation. It is also important to realize that the cardiac catheterization lab is not the only place where patients receive radiation (Fig. 1.1).[6] Other factors to consider include which, if any, other tests the patients have received prior to coming to the catheterization lab (i.e., nuclear stress test, computed tomography [CT] angiogram, etc.) and how much radiation they have been exposed to for those studies (Table 1.1).

Each catheterization lab is set up differently, but they are all designed with the C-arm and floating patient table as the main focus of the room. The C-arm consists of two components, a radiation source and an image receptor (intensifiers on older systems or flat-panel detectors on modern units). X-ray films are produced when energy is applied to convert atoms into high-energy x-ray photons and directed in a beam from the generator, through the patient, and then detected in an image intensifier or flat-panel detector above the patient. The radiation source provides the most risk to the operator, patient, and staff. The image intensifier or flat-panel detector captures radiation and converts it into an image usable for immediate viewing on the monitor and able to be stored on a mainframe for later review. An object can be seen on an x-ray image if

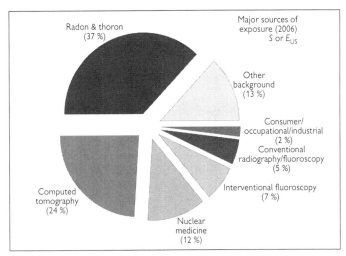

Figure 1.1 Major sources of exposure. Fifty percent of all radiation that individuals are exposed to comes from human-made sources of radiation, with the majority of those related to medical imaging. Reprinted with permission of the National Council on Radiation Protection and Measurements, http://NCRPonline.org.

Table 1.1 Relative radiation doses in medical imaging

Examination	Representative Effective Dose Value (mSv)	Range of Reported Effective Dose Values (mSv)	Administered Activity (MBq)
Chest x-ray PA and lateral	0.1	0.05–0.24	NA
CT chest	7	4–18	NA
CT abdominal	8	4–25	NA
CT pelvis	6	3–10	NA
Coronary calcium CT*	3	1–12	NA
Coronary CT angiogram[†]	16	5–32	NA
64-Slice coronary CTA[‡]			
Without tube current modulation	15	12–18	NA
With tube current modulation	9	8–18	NA
Dual-source coronary CTA[‡]			
With tube current modulation	. 13	6–17	NA
Prospectively triggered coronary CTA[‡]	3	2–4	NA
Diagnostic invasive coronary angiogram	7	2–16	NA
Percutaneous coronary intervention or radiofrequency ablation	15	7–57	NA
Myocardial perfusion study			
Sestamibi (1-day) stress/rest	9	—	1100
Thallium stress/rest	41	—	185
F-18 FDG	14	—	740
Rubidium-82	5	—	1480

* Data combine prospectively triggered and retrospectively gated protocols. The Writing Group estimates the representative effective dose estimate to be approximately 1 mSv for prospectively triggered coronary calcium CT scans and 3 mSv for retrospectively gated scans.

† Includes data published between 1980 and 2007. Dose data may not reflect newest scanners and protocols.

‡ 64-Slice multidetector-row CT and dual-source CT studies published since 2005 only; data include a survey of the literature by the Writing Group.

PA, poseteroanterior; CTA, CT angiography; FDG, flurodeoxyglucose; NA, not applicable.

Source: Gerber, TC, et al. *Circulation* 2009;119:1056-1065, American Heart Association, Inc.

its x-ray absorbance is different from that of surrounding structures. Iodinated contrast agents effectively assure this absorbance difference between the blood vessels and surrounding tissues to allow for the performance of selective coronary angiography.

The radiation source and image receptor have multiple parts that help to determine the amount of radiation emitted from the source, including beam collimators, lead shields, and x-ray brightness detectors, which, via feedback loops, determine how much energy is needed to generate an acceptable image. Flat-panel detectors use a charge-coupled device (CCD) visible light detector to generate the image directly from the original light emission without the modifications required by the older image intensifiers. This CCD is also able to use the digital output signal level to guide the amount of radiation exposure to generate interpretable images. X-ray images are affected by x-ray beam power, filtration, scattered radiation, and image noise. Increasing beam power by increasing kVp will decrease its tissue absorption and allow penetration of denser body parts. However, increasing kVp will also decrease beam modulation and image contrast, decreasing the relative absorption differences between tissues. Increasing electrical power applied (mA) will increase the number of x-ray photons that penetrate the patient. This will effectively decrease image noise at the cost of higher overall patient and operator exposure. Basic descriptors of relative radiation quantities are described in Table 1.2.

Training to limit risk from x-ray radiation centers around the concept of ALARA (as low as reasonably achievable). Basically stated, operator and patient risk is limited by reducing exposure levels to x-ray radiation to the bare minimum necessary to perform the test. Several methods exist to minimize radiation exposure, and they revolve around three major factors: time, distance, and shielding.

Limiting the total time using fluoroscopy and cineangiography will translate into fewer x-rays that will be emitted from the radiation source, and this will decrease both the patient's and staff's exposure to radiation. There are two basic modes of imaging within the catheterization lab that must be considered with respect to x-ray radiation: fluoroscopy and cineangiography. Operators should be cognizant of the fact that cineangiography utilizes 10–15 times the amount of radiation per frame as regular imaging, and therefore the number of cineangiographic images obtained should be kept to the minimum number needed to accurately diagnose and treat the problem. Fluoroscopy, although lower in total x-ray scatter radiation, has a greater potential for abuse, as operators have a tendency to stay on the peddle for prolonged periods of time. Although a poor surrogate for the actual amount of radiation emitted and absorbed, the fluoroscopy time can help gauge how much radiation exposure the patient and staff have received and possibly help to determine stopping places in nonemergent cases. Most modern catheterization labs utilize "pulsed fluoroscopy" modes, in which the x-rays are not sent out continuously, but rather are pulsed to lower the total radiation emitted. The slower the pulse rate, the lower the exposure.

Table 1.2 Relative radiation quantities

Quantity	Units of Measurement	What It Is	What It Measures	Why It's Useful	Conversion between Old and New Units
Absorbed dose	gray (Gy) or milligray (mGy) [rad or millirad (mrad)]	The amount of energy locally deposited in tissue per unit mass of tissue	Measures concentration of energy deposition in tissue	Assesses the potential biological risk to that specific tissue	1 rad = 10 mGy
Effective dose	sievert (Sv) or millisievert (mSv) [rem or millirem (mrem)]	An attributed whole-body dose that produces the same whole-person stochastic risk as an absorbed dose to a limited portion of the body	Converts any localized absorbed or equivalent dose to a whole-body risk factor	Permits comparison of risks among several exposed individuals, even though the doses might be delivered to different sets of organs in these individuals	1 rem = 10 mSv
Air kerma*	gray (Gy) or milligray (mGy) [rad or millirad (mrad)]	The sum of initial kinetic energies of all charged particles liberated by the x-rays per mass of air	Measures amount of radiation at a point in space	Assesses the level of hazard at the specified location†	1 rad = 10 mGy
Exposure	millicoulomb·kr⁻¹ [roentgen (R) or milliroentgen (mR)]	The total charge of ions of one sign produced by the radiation per unit mass of air	Measures amount of radiation at a point in space	Assess the level of hazard at the specified location†	1 millicoulomb·kgr⁻¹ 4 Roentgen (R)

Table 1.2 Continued

Quantity	Units of Measurement	What It Is	What It Measures	Why It's Useful	Conversion between Old and New Units
Equivalent dose‡	sievert (Sv) or millisievert (mSv) [rem or millirem (mrem)]	A dose quantity that factors in the relative biological damage caused by different types of radiations	Provides a relative dose that accounts for increased biological damage from some types of radiations	This is the most common unit used to measure radiation risk to specific tissues for radiation protection of personnel‡	1 rem = 10 mSv

* Air kerma can be presented in two separate ways. Incident air kerma is the kerma to air from an incident x-ray beam measured on the central beam axis at the position of the patient and excludes backscattered radiation. Entrance surface air kerma is the kerma to air from an incident x-ray beam measured on the central beam axis at the position of the patient with backscattered radiation included. The two may differ from each other by up to about 40%.

† Exposure and air kerma are both used for the same purpose. Exposure used to be the most common measure, but with the switch to international units, air kerma is the preferred unit.

‡ For x-rays, gamma rays, and electrons, there is no difference between absorbed dose and equivalent dose, i.e., 1 mGy = 1 mSv. This is not the case for neutrons and alpha particles, but these radiation types are not relevant to x-ray exposure. The important issue is that cardiologists recognize that for their interests there is no practical difference between a measurement of mGy and that of mSv.

Reprinted from Hirshfeld JW, Balter S, Brinker JA, et al. (2004). ACCF/AHA/HRS/SCAI clinical competence statement on optimizing patient safety and image quality in fluoroscopically guided invasive cardiovascular procedures: a report of the American College of Cardiology/American Heart Association/American College of Physicians Task Force on Clinical Competence (ACCF/AHA/HRS/SCAI Writing Committee to Develop a Clinical Competence Statement on Fluoroscopy). *Journal of the American College of Cardiology*, 44:2259-2282. Copyright © 2004 American College of Cardiology Foundation. With permission from Elsevier.

The magnification utilized during imaging also affects the amount of radiation emitted, with 5-inch (13-cm) modes requiring the greatest amount of radiation to reduce image noise seen at these greater degrees of magnification. Imaging on a 9-inch (22-centimeter) setting will help to reduce the amount of radiation emitted, as opposed to using smaller imaging formats (i.e., 5-inch). Reducing the frame rate at which patients are imaged will also help to reduce the radiation exposure to the patients; if possible, operators should aim for 7.5–15 frames per second. Other opportunities to decrease the radiation exposure by utilizing equipment features are available for the operator. Collimation can be set up to "frame" the area of interest within the picture, decreasing the impact of the air-filled lung fields and thereby decreasing the overall energy necessary to create diagnostic images. Likewise, the ability to store fluoroscopically derived images and decreased cineangiographic runs are now commonplace in most labs.

Distance relates to radiation exposure by the inverse square law, which is shown in the following equation: Radiation exposure $= 1/\text{distance}^2$. This suggests that the greater distance the operator is from the radiation source, the lower the amount of radiation he or she will be exposed to during the procedure. Operators should therefore get their catheters/equipment into place and stand back as far as they can from the radiation source while performing fluoroscopy and cineangiograms. Based upon the way radiation is emitted from the source, operators should also try to work in angiographic views that maximize the distance between themselves and the radiation source (Table 1.3). Another distance that is important to keep in mind is the distance between the image receptor and the radiation source. Keeping the image intensifier or flat-panel detector as close to the patient as possible will minimize both the radiation dose and scatter.

Shielding is yet another protective mechanism. Because it is largely based upon lead materials, shielding is often limited by weight. The lead aprons worn in the past were both heavy and cumbersome; several previous operators are currently experiencing orthopedic (specifically spine) injuries from wearing lead for multiple decades.[7] Nearly half of the physicians surveyed in a SCAI survey had experienced spine problems, compared with an incidence of 27.4% in the average American population.[8] This has caused significant morbidity and shortened the careers of many interventionalists. Newer, "lighter lead" protective gear will hopefully help to reduce these ailments, but it will still be very important to limit the amount of time wearing leaded equipment and optimizing posture to further minimize risk (wearers of protective gear that uses lead substitutes must ensure that they are getting the same risk-reduction levels with whatever substance is being used). Leaded glasses are important to reduce eye exposure and prevent cataract formation.[7] Making proper utilization of shielding within the lab is also important to reduced exposure. All labs should have a lead skirt that hangs off of the side of the table, and this should be pulled out against the operator's left hip to protect against under-table radiation scatter.

Table 1.3 Radiation scatter and image view	
Angiographic View	Waist-level Scatter (mR/hr)
AP	34
RAO 30	20
LAO 30	103
Lateral	204

A ceiling-mounted shield should be utilized to abut against the patient and be placed between the above-table detector and the operator to protect against over-table scatter. Portable leaded shielding can also be utilized for procedures that force the operator to be positioned closer to the radiation source.

The methods to measure how much radiation exposure a patient receives are not ideal, given that these are not exact measures, but instead are estimations based on models.[1] The interventional reference point (IRP) is an approximation of the dose received at the skin when the heart is used as the focus of the imaging procedure, and it is measured in air kerma. The dose-area product (DAP) is the air kerma multiplied by the x-ray beam cross-sectional area at the point of measurement, and it is considered to be a representation of the total amount of radiation administered to the patient. The DAP is usually measured from an ionization chamber in the x-ray tube or can be estimated based upon generator and collimator settings. Some believe that DAP can used to estimate stochastic risks from x-ray procedures. The IRP and DAP may be inaccurate when cranial or caudal views are the primary working views during the procedure.

Some illnesses may predispose patients to a higher risk of radiation-induced skin damage. Hyperthyroidism, diabetes mellitus, ataxia telangiectasia, and collagen vascular diseases (especially scleroderma, discoid lupus, and mixed connective tissue disease) all increase the patient's risk.[1] These patients may benefit from limited radiation exposure, and diligence should be utilized to assess for skin breakdown during clinic follow-up after their procedures.

Fetal exposure to radiation can be catastrophic and, in addition to the dose received, the stage of gestation plays a role in long-term effects (Table 1.4). Major consequences to the fetus include growth retardation, malformation, and central nervous system defects, with childhood leukemia also being a risk. Fluoroscopic procedures performed in pregnancy are not absolutely contraindicated because the amount of radiation that the fetus is exposed to is small; nonetheless, special care and consultation with a radiation safety officer are recommended to help reduce risk to its absolute minimum.[9] According to the Nuclear Regulatory Commission's dose limits, women who work in the catheterization or electrophysiology labs can choose not to declare their pregnancy and continue to work with the same radiation dose limitations as usual

Table 1.4 Maximum annual occupational dose limits	
Maximum Annual Occupational Dose Limits	mRem
Whole body	5,000
Extremities	50,000
Skin	50,000
Individual organs	50,000
Lens of the eye	15,000
Fetus (during the entire gestational period)	500
Minors (<18 years) working with radioactive materials	500
Individuals in the general public	100
Modified from http://www.nrc.gov/reading-rm/doc-collections/cfr/part020/part020-1201.html	

(5 Rem/year).[9] If she declares her pregnancy, the worker will be restricted to 500 mRem for the entire length of the gestation period to minimize risk. The current recommendations for radiation protection in pregnant women are summarized in Table 1.5.

Summary

Exposure to radiation is inherent in several cardiac imaging techniques and is particularly relevant for the interventional cardiologist. The primary operator should try to minimize exposure to him- or herself, catheterization lab personnel, and the patient by using shielding, the lowest possible dose of radiation, and appropriate collimation.

Practical Pearls

- Overall goal is to limit patient and operator radiation exposure by:
  - Increasing distance away from source of radiation
  - Limiting total fluoroscopic time and cineangiographic runs
  - Utilizing all possible shielding and barriers

Contrast Agents in the Catheterization Lab

Iodinated contrast agents have progressively evolved since their first successful intravascular use in the 1950s. All modern contrast agents are based upon iodine, because of its ability to delineate vascular structures throughout the body when used with x-ray imaging systems. Contrast agents are differentiated by iodine concentration, osmolality, and ionicity (Table 1.6). Original contrast agents are high-osmolar formulations and are poorly tolerated secondary to intense flushing, myocardial depression, and ventricular arrhythmia with injection. These agents are ratio-1.5 ionic compounds, as they have three atoms of iodine for every two ions. In addition to the side effects just listed, these agents

Table 1.5 Radiation safety during pregnancy

Exposure

1. Pregnant women should be able to safely perform all duties provided that strict attention is paid to exposure limits.

2. Exposure should not exceed 0.5 rem (5 mSv) over entire pregnancy or 0.05 rem (0.5 mSv) in any single month.

3. Consider reducing exposure during gestational weeks 8–15 to reduce risk of fetal mental retardation.

Shielding

1. Use same precautions as all operators.

2. Use maternity aprons.

3. Other shielding options are not recommended, such as:

    —lead underwear

    —double aprons, which may cause imbalance and injury

4. Inspect lead aprons fluoroscopically on a monthly basis.

Monitoring

1. Two film badges should be worn in the catheterization or electrophysiology laboratory:

    —one at neck outside of lead

    —one at waist inside of lead

2. In the nuclear laboratory, two film badges should be worn:

    —one at chest level

    —one at waist level (if lead is worn, only the waist badge is worn under lead)

3. Badges should be monitored monthly, although weekly is ideal.

4. Women in the catheterization and electrophysiology laboratories, particularly with a personal exposure history for the current year >0.1 rem, should monitor exposure on a case-by-case basis using a pocket ionization chamber and maintain a record of readings; this does not substitute for a badge that monitors cumulative exposure.

Counseling

1. Every woman has the prerogative to choose between continuing her professional activities within exposure recommendations listed above or restricting them during all or part of her pregnancy.

2. Such decisions should be based on knowledge of risks, monitoring options and shielding techniques, and, most important, personal history of radiation exposures.

3. Every woman should have the opportunity to discuss these issues privately and confidentially with an unbiased knowledgeable individual (e.g., a radiation safety officer). At the time the pregnancy is declared, the woman and radiation safety officer will review previous exposure records, evaluate monthly exposure history, and plan activities and monitoring during the pregnancy.

4. Cardiology laboratory directors should recognize that pregnancy by itself should not limit activities in the laboratory but should support female personnel who choose to reduce their exposure by limiting their radiation-related activities.

Reprinted from Limacher MC, Douglas PC, Germano G, et al. Radiation safety in the practice of cardiology. *J Am Coll Cardiol*. 1998;31:892-913, With permission from Elsevier.

Table 1.6 Characteristics of iodinated contrast agents

Type		Iodine (mg/mL)	Osmolality (mOsm/kg)	Viscosity @ 37°C	Trade Name (Brand Name)
High-osmolar	Ratio 1.5 (3:2)	370	2076	8.4	Diatrizoate (Hypaque, Renografin)
High-osmolar	Ratio 1.5 (3:2)	325	1797	28	Iothalmate (Conray)
Low-osmolar ionic dimer	Ratio 3 (6:2)	320	600	7.5	Ioxaglate (Hexabrix)
Low-osmolar nonionic	Ratio 3 (3:1)	370	796	9.4	Iopamidol (Isovue)
Low-osmolar nonionic	Ratio 3 (3:1)	350	844	10.4	Iohexol (Omnipaque)
Low-osmolar nonionic	Ratio 3 (3:1)	350	792	9.0	Ioversol (Optiray)
Iso-osmolar nonionic dimer	Ratio 6 (6:1)	320	290	11.8	Iodixanol (Visipaque)

also have very high osmolarity (approximately 1,500–2,075 mOsm/kg), which is severalfold (>5 times) higher than blood and could contribute to an overall volume imbalance in patients predisposed to such a condition (i.e., congestive heart failure, renal insufficiency).

The second generation of contrast agents did not come into practice until almost 30 years after the introduction of the high-osmolar agents. The ratio-3 agents are considered low-osmolar, given that their osmolarity is only twice that of blood. These agents have three atoms of iodine for every one ion or molecule in the structure. There are two subgroups, one being an ionic dimer and the other a nonionic dimer. Because of their lower tonicity, these agents produce fewer side effects; they have become the staple of several catheterization labs throughout the country, based upon their improved side-effect profile (compared to first-generation agents) and their affordable cost (compared to third-generation agents).

The most recent contrast formulation to reach the market is a ratio-6 non-ionic dimeric compound. This is the only iso-osmolar contrast agent, and it actually requires the addition of sodium and calcium chloride to increase the osmolarity to a level similar to blood. The major benefit of this agent lies in the even further reduction of minor allergic reactions and some of the side effects, such as flushing. To date, there is only one randomized trial showing superiority of this ratio-6 agent to the nonionic low-osmolar compounds with regards to the incidence of nephrotoxicity.[10] Most trials have shown no significant difference in the development of nephrotoxicity between various agents, and other factors such as minimizing contrast use and prehydration with normal saline are more important aspects in reducing risk.[11–12] It is of the utmost importance that the operator monitor how much contrast is utilized during a procedure and, in special patient populations (i.e., diabetics, the elderly, heart failure with elevated EDP, and those with renal insufficiency), use low- or iso-osmolar agents to further reduce risk and avoid invasive procedures altogether unless absolutely necessary.

Contrast agents are associated with adverse events that demand particular focus in that their treatment and/or prevention are important elements of clinical practice in the catheterization lab. Allergic reactions to iodinated contrast agents complicate fewer than 1% of all catheterizations but can be lethal if not promptly recognized and treated. The reaction is technically anaphylactoid in nature, as it involves mast cell degranulation and histamine release but does not require previous exposure to contrast. Clinical manifestations of anaphylactoid contrast reactions include everything from erythremia and urticaria to hemodynamic collapse and shock. Treatment for anaphylactoid reactions and prevention of subsequent reactions are summarized in Table 1.7. Successful treatment when these reactions occur centers on prompt diagnosis and immediate therapy.

The more common complication of contrast administration is contrast-associated nephropathy. It is most frequently defined as an increase in serum creatinine of 25% or 0.5 mg/dL and occurs in 1%–15% of patients receiving contrast.[13–14] Various patient-related risk factors have been shown to contribute significantly to the development of contrast nephropathy, and risk scores to predict its occurrence have been developed (Fig. 1.2).[15] This type of risk prediction identifies patients in whom measures should be adopted to try to decrease their risk of developing nephropathy.

Reducing the incidence of contrast-related nephropathy centers around assuring adequate volume status for the patient and limiting the total amount of contrast administered. Total contrast dose has been shown to contribute to this complication, and various authors have supported a threshold limit for at-risk patients.[16] Many strategies (including medications) have been studied as potential paths that could reduce contrast-related nephropathy, and these are summarized in Table 1.8. For the most part, pharmacologic agents have been

Table 1.7 Management of contrast reactions		
Contrast Reaction Prophylaxis	Preprocedure	Diphenhydramine 50 mg; prednisone 50 mg: at least 2 doses 12 hours and 1–4 hours prior to procedure
Anaphalactoid Treatment	Mild Reaction (urticaria)	Diphenhydramine 25–5 mg IV
	Bronchospasm	Diphenhydramine 50 mg IV; hydrocortisone 200–400 mg IV, albuterol inhaler (consider epinephrine SQ 0.3 cc of 1:1,000, repeat up to 1 cc for severe reactions)
	Hypotension/Shock	IV epinephrine 1:10,000) 0.1 mg IV slowly over 5 minutes; hydrocortisone 400 mg; diphenhydramine 50–100 mg IV; dopamine; ACLS support

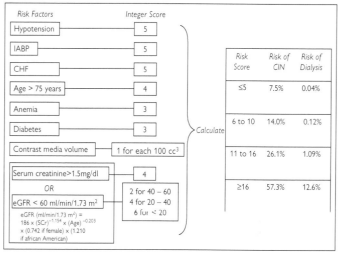

Figure 1.2 **Risk factors**. Adapted with permission from Mehran R, Aymong ED, Nikolsky E, et al. A simple risk score for prediction of contrast-induced nephropathy after percutaneous coronary intervention. Development and initial validation. *J Am Coll Cardiol*. 2004; 44:1393-1399.

Table 1.8 Summary of strategies to reduce contrast-induced nephropathy

Strategy	Relative Benefit
Eliminate/hold administering other potentially nephrotoxic agents (e.g., ACE-inhibitor or NSAID)	+/–
Hydration with 0.9% normal saline pre and post contrast administration	+++
Hydration with sodium bicarbonate	+
Limit the overall amount of injected contrast (volume of contrast/CrCl >3.7)	+++
N-acetylcysteine	+/–
Furosemide	–
Mannitol	–
Fenoldopam	–
Dopamine	–
ACE, angiotensin-converting enzyme; NSAID, nonsteroidal anti-inflammatory drug; CrCl, creatinine clearance.	

ineffective at dramatically reducing any patient's risk of nephropathy, and recommendations continue to stress that fluid administration to assure adequate intravascular volume is the most important preventative measure.

Summary

Contrast injection is an integral part of diagnostic and interventional cardiology. Appropriate knowledge of the types of available contrast agents is important for clinicians. Every effort should be made to minimize the amount of contrast used during a procedure and ascertain that patients are adequately hydrated before the procedure. Severe contrast reactions, although rare, need to be identified early and treated aggressively to avoid fatality. Despite aggressive treatment, deaths have occurred with severe contrast reaction.

Practical Pearls

- Current practice principally utilizes low-osmolar nonionic or iso-osmolar nonionic agents.
- Risk factors associated with contrast nephropathy principally include preexisting renal disease and diabetes.
- Anaphylactoid reactions require prompt treatment with diphenhydramine, epinephrine, and hydrocortisone.

References

1. Hirshfeld JW, Balter S, Brinker JA, et al. ACCF/AHA/HRS/SCAI Clinical competence statement on physician knowledge to optimize patient safety and image quality in fluoroscopically guided invasive cardiovascular procedures: a report of the American College of Cardiology Foundation/American Heart Association/ American College of Physicians Task Force on Clinical Competence and Training. *Circulation.* 2005;111:511-532.

2. Gerber TC, Carr JJ, Arai AE, et al. Ionizing radiation in cardiac imaging: a science advisory from the American Heart Association Committee on Cardiac Imaging of the Council on Clinical Cardiology and Committee on Cardiovascular Imaging and Intervention of the Council on Cardiovascular Radiology and Intervention. *Circulation.* 2009;119:1056-1065.

3. United Nations Scientific Committee on the Effects of Atomic Radiation. *Sources and effects of ionizing radiation.* New York: United Nations; 2000. Accessed May 18, 2009 at http://www.unscear.org/unscear/en/publications/2000_2.html

4. Committee to Assess Health Risks from Exposure to Low Levels of Ionizing Radiation, Board on Radiation Effects Research Division on Earth and Life Studies, National Research Council of the National Academies. *Health risks from exposure to low levels of ionizing radiation: BEIR VII-Phase 2.* Washington, DC: National Academies Press, 2006.

5. National Council on Radiation Protection and Measurements. *Report 94. Exposure of the population in the United States and Canada from natural background radiation.* Bethesda, MD: National Council on Radiation Protection and Measurements, 1988.

6. National Council on Radiation Protection and Measurements. *Report 100. Exposure of the U.S. population from diagnostic medical radiation.* Bethesda, MD: National Council on Radiation Protection and Measurements; 1989.

7. Klein LW, Miller DL, Balter S, et al. Occupational health hazards in the interventional laboratory: time for a safer environment. *Cath Cardiovasc Intervent.* 2009;73:432-438.

8. Goldstein JA, Balter S, Cowley M, et al. Occupational hazards of interventional cardiologists: prevalence of orthopedic health problems in contemporary practice. *Cath Cardiovasc Intervent.* 2004;63:407-411.

9. United States Nuclear Regulatory Commission. Conditions requiring individual monitoring of external and internal occupational dose. 1998. Accessed May 1, 2009 at http://www.nrc.gov/reading-rm/doc-collections/cfr/part020/part020-1502.html

10. Aspelin P, Aubry P, Fransson S, et al. Nephrotoxic effects in high-risk patients undergoing angiography. *N Eng J Med.* 2003;348:491-499.

11. McCullough PA, Bertrand ME, Brinker JA, Stacul F. A meta-analysis of the renal safety of isosmolar iodixanol compared with low-osmolal contrast media. *J Am Coll Cardiol.* 2006;48:692-699.

12. Schweiger MJ, Chambers CE, Davidson CJ, et al. Prevention of contrast induced nephropathy: recommendations for the high risk patient undergoing cardiovascular procedures. *Cath Cardiovasc Intervent.* 2007;69:135-140.

13. Levy EM, Viscoli CM, Howritz RI. The effect of acute renal failure on mortality. A cohort analysis. *JAMA.* 1996;275:1489-1494.

14. Best PJ, Lennon R, Ting HH, et al. The impact of renal insufficiency on clinical outcomes in patients undergoing percutaneous coronary interventions. *J Am Coll Cardiol.* 2002;39:1113-1119.

15. Mehran R, Aymong ED, Nikolsky E, et al. A simple risk score for prediction of contrast-induced nephropathy after percutaneous coronary intervention. Development and initial validation. *J Am Coll Cardiol.* 2004;44:1393-1399.

16. Kane GC, Doyle BJ, Lerman A, et al. Ultra-low contrast volumes reduce rates of contrast-induced nephropathy in patients with chronic kidney disease undergoing coronary angiography. *J Am Coll Cardiol.* 2008;51:89-90.

Chapter 2

Antiplatelets, Antithrombotics, Vasodilators, and Vasopressors

Calvin Choi and Mike Sarkees

Acute coronary syndrome (ACS), which is defined as acute myocardial infarction (MI) or unstable angina, accounts for over 1.5 million annual hospitalizations in the United States.[1] More than 1.2 million percutaneous coronary interventions (PCIs) are performed annually,[1] making this procedure the cornerstone of modern cardiovascular revascularization, and it has advanced by leaps and bounds since its inception. In addition to the technical aspects of PCI, adjunct pharmacotherapy has evolved over the years, and it has a tremendous impact on paradigm, efficacy, and clinical outcome. In this chapter, major adjunct pharmacotherapy for PCI (antiplatelet agents, antithrombin agents, intracoronary agents, and vasopressors) will be reviewed.

Antiplatelets

Endothelial injury, in particular, atherosclerotic plaque rupture, results in adhesion, activation, and aggregation of platelets, which in turn cause flow-limiting thrombus.[2] As such, antiplatelet therapy (Table 2.1) plays a key role in adjunct pharmacotherapy for PCI during elective and ACS situations.

Aspirin

Aspirin irreversibly inactivates cyclooxygenase (COX), with subsequent inhibition of thromboxane A_2 production for the life of the platelet.[2] Thromboxane A_2 propagates platelet activation, and it is a potent vasoconstrictor.[2]

The America College of Cardiology and American Heart Association (ACC/AHA) recommends initiation and indefinite continuation of aspirin therapy when coronary artery disease, and especially ACS, is suspected in the absence of contraindications.[3]

Aspirin (325 mg) should be administered as soon as possible prior to PCI.[4] For those patients who are initially unable to tolerate oral therapy, aspirin can be administered per rectum.

Table 2.1 Antiplatelet agents

	Loading Dose	Maintenance
Aspirin	• 325 mg	• BMS: 162–325 mg/day for at least 1 month then 75–162 mg/day indefinitely • DES: 162–325 mg/day for at least 3–6 months (3 and 6 months for sirolimus and paclitaxel stents, respectively) then 75–162 mg/day indefinitely
Clopidogrel	• 300–600 mg • 300 mg if PCI performed within 12–24 hours of fibrolytic therapy	• BMS: 75 mg/day for at least 1 month, ideally 1 year • DES: 75 mg/day for at least 1 year
Ticlopidine	• 500 mg	• 250 mg twice daily
Prasugrel	• 60 mg	• 10 mg once daily • 5 mg/day for high-risk patients with weight <60 kg and/or age >75 years
Ticagrelor	• 180 mg	• 90 mg twice daily
Glycoprotein IIb/IIIa inhibitor		
Abciximab	• 0.25 mg/kg	• 0.125 mcg/kg/min (maximum 10 mcg/min) for 12 hours post PCI
Eptifibatide	• 180 mcg/kg followed by another 180 mcg/kg in 10 minutes • Maximum 22.6 mg/bolus	• 2 mcg/kg/min (maximum 242 mcg/min) for 18–24 hours post PCI • For CrCl <50 mL/min, 1 mcg/kg/min
Tirofiban	• 0.4 mcg/kg/min for 30 minutes	• 0.1 mcg/kg/min for 18–24 hours post PCI • For CrCl <30 mL/min, 0.05 mcg/kg/min
Cilostazol		• 100 mg twice daily

Clopidogrel

Clopidogrel is a thienopyridine that inhibits adenosine diphosphate (ADP)-mediated platelet aggregation by irreversibly binding the ADP P_2Y receptor.[5] Clopidogrel is a prodrug that requires conversion to an active metabolite before binding to the ADP P_2Y receptor to confer its antiplatelet activity.[5]

The ACC/AHA guidelines recommend dual antiplatelet therapy (clopidogrel and aspirin), with a loading dose of clopidogrel for patients with ACS undergoing PCI.[3,4] A loading dose of 300–600 mg is recommended prior to PCI.[5] If PCI is planned within 12–24 hours after fibrolytic therapy, a 300 mg loading dose of clopidogrel can be considered.[4]

For ACS patients who receive medical therapy without PCI, and for those who receive a bare metal stent (BMS), clopidogrel 75 mg/day is recommended for at least 1 month; however, 1 year of therapy is considered optimal.[3] For patients who receive a drug-eluting stent (DES), clopidogrel 75 mg/day for at least 1 year is recommended.[3] For patients undergoing coronary artery bypass grafting (CABG), clopidogrel should be withheld at least 5 days prior to the surgery.[6]

Ticlopidine

Ticlopidine is an irreversible platelet ADP receptor inhibitor.[7] Ticlopidine therapy has been largely abandoned in clinical practice and replaced by clopidogrel, due to its potential adverse hematological reactions, including neutropenia, agranulocytosis, thrombotic thrombocytopenic purpura, and aplastic anemia.

Ticlopidine is administered as a 500 mg loading dose followed by 250 mg twice daily.[7] In case of clopidogrel allergy, ticlopidine therapy may be considered. Hematological adverse reactions tend to occur within the first few weeks of initiation of therapy. As such, hematological adverse reactions should be monitored closely during the first 3 months of use.

Prasugrel

Prasugrel, like clopidogrel, is a thienopyridine that inhibits ADP-mediated platelet aggregation by irreversibly binding the ADP P_2Y receptor.[8] It also is a prodrug that requires conversion to an active metabolite before binding to the ADP P_2Y receptor to confer its antiplatelet activity.[8]

When compared with clopidogrel (300 mg load and 75 mg/day), prasugrel reduced the composite of death from cardiovascular causes, nonfatal MI, or nonfatal stroke; however, it increased the risk of bleeding.[8]

Prasugrel is administered as a loading dose of 60 mg within 1 hour of the completion of PCI, followed by a 10 mg/day maintenance dose for the patients with ACS with or without ST segment elevation undergoing PCI.[8] Prasugrel is contraindicated in patients with a history of stroke or in need of an urgent surgery, including CABG surgery.[8] Prasugrel is generally not recommended for patients who weigh less than 60 kg and/or are older than 75 years. However, for high-risk patients (diabetes and/or previous MI), the drug dosage may be reduced to 5 mg/day.[8]

Novel Antiplatelet Agents

Ticagrelor is a short-acting ADP P_2Y receptor inhibitor that showed promising results in a recent trial.[9] When compared with clopidogrel, ticagrelor significantly reduced the composite of death from vascular causes, MI, or stroke in patients with ACS with or without ST segment elevation.[9] Ticagrelor is administered as a loading dose of 180 mg followed by 90 mg twice daily.[9]

The main advantage of ticagrelor, when compared with currently available ADP P_2Y receptor inhibitors, is that it is functionally reversible once the effect of the drug has worn off. Ticagrelor is currently being studied in clinical trials but is not yet available for commercial use.

Glycoprotein IIb/IIIa Inhibitors

Glycogen IIb/IIIa inhibitors bind to fibrinogen receptors and thus prevent platelet aggregation. Because of the risk for profound thrombocytopenia, the platelet count should be monitored after glycogen IIb/IIIa inhibitor infusion.

The ACC/AHA guideline indicates that the addition of glycoprotein IIb//IIIa inhibitor (eptifibatide or tirofiban) is reasonable for patients with ACS in the absence of ST segment elevation MI who develop recurrent angina despite dual antiplatelet and anticoagulation therapy or who are already on dual antiplatelet therapy and will be undergoing PCI.[3] However, recent studies indicate that routine upstream use of IIb/IIIa inhibitor may increase the risk of bleeding, and clinical benefit may not be as robust as previously thought.[10, 11]

Abciximab is a chimeric human mouse monoclonal antibody that is indicated for PCI in conjunction with an antithrombin agent. Abciximab is administered as 0.25 mg/kg bolus prior to initiation of PCI, followed by continuous infusion at 0.125 µg/kg/min (maximum 10 µg/min) for 12 hours post PCI.[12]

Eptifibatide is a cyclic heptapeptide used in conjunction with an antithrombin agent during PCI. Eptifibatide is administered as a bolus, 180 µg/kg (maximum 22.6 mg) followed by another bolus 180 µg/kg 10 minutes after the initial bolus, with a 2 µg/kg/min (maximum 242 µg/min) infusion after the first bolus for 18–24 hours post PCI.[13] For creatinine clearance less than 50 ml /min, bolus dose of 180 µg/kg is administered once, then a continuous infusion is reduced to 1 µg/kg/min.[13]

Tirofiban is given as a bolus dose of 0.4 µg/kg/min for 30 minutes, followed by 0.1 µg/kg/min for 18–24 hours of continuous infusion post PCI.[14] For creatinine clearance of less than 30 mL/min, the rate of infusion is reduced by 50%.[14]

Cilostazol

Cilostazol is a phosphodiesterase III inhibitor that inhibits platelet adhesion. Because of its association with increased mortality, cilostazol is contraindicated in congestive heart failure of any severity.

There is evidence to suggest that triple antiplatelet therapy—the addition of cilostazol to aspirin and clopidogrel or ticlopidine—may reduce the incidence of stent thrombosis and restenosis.[15] Cilostazol is administered 100 mg twice daily.

Antithrombotics

Despite potent antiplatelet therapy, patients with ACS are at risk for adverse ischemic events. As part of the platelet adhesion, activation, and aggregation continuum, clotting factors contribute to flow-limiting thrombus, resulting in vessel obstruction with subsequent ACS; antithrombotics reduce this risk (Table 2.2).

Unfractionated Heparin

Unfractionated heparin potentiates protease inhibitor antithrombin, which inactivates clotting factors Xa and IIa.[3]

Heparin is given as an initial bolus of 60 units/kg (maximum 4,000 units) followed by 12 units/kg/hr (maximum 1,000 units/hr).[3] When used in conjunction with a glycoprotein IIb/IIa during PCI, the goal-activated clotting time should be 200–250 seconds; without it, 250–300 seconds by HemoTec or 300–350 seconds by Hemochron.[3]

Heparin dose response is highly variable, and it can cause heparin-induced thrombocytopenia, as well as rebound hypercoagulable state. Heparin should

Table 2.2 Antithrombotics

	Loading Dose	Maintenance
Unfractionated Heparin	• 60 units/kg • Maximum 4,000 units	• 12 units/kg/hr • ACT 200–250 seconds when used in conjunction with glycoprotein IIb/IIa inhibitor • Without glycoprotein IIb/IIIa inhibitor, 250–300 or 300–350 seconds by HemoTec or Hemochron, respectively
LMWH*	• STEMI: 30 mg IV bolus • For age >75 years, no bolus • 0.3 mg/kg IV bolus if last SC dose was more than 8 hours before PCI	• STEMI or NSTEMI: 1 mg/kg SC every 12 hours • For CrCl <30 mL/min, SC every 24 hours • For age >75 years, 0.75 mg/kg every 12 hours
Bivalirudin	• 0.75 mg/kg without previous bolus • 0.5 mg/kg bolus just prior to PCI if initial medical therapy began with a 0.1 mg/kg bolus followed by 0.25 mg/kg/hr	• 1.75 mg/kg/hr up to 4 hours during PCI • For CrCl <30 mL/min, 1 mg/kg/hr
Fondaparinux*	• STEMI: 2.5 mg IV • Use in conjunction with 50–60 units/kg IV heparin bolus during PCI	• STEMI or NSTEMI: 2.5 mg SC daily • Contraindicated for CrCl <30 mL/minute

*Loading and maintenance dosages for LMWH and fondaparinux are for initial medical therapy.

STEMI, ST elevation myocardial infarction; ACT, activated clotting time; PCI, percutaneous coronary intervention; NSTEMI, non-ST elevation myocardial infarction; CrCl, creatinine clearance.

ACT, activated clotting time; BMS, bare metal stent; CrCl, creatinine clearance; DES, drug eluting stent; IC, intracoronary; IV, intravenous; LMWH, low molecular weight heparin; NSTEMI, non ST segment elevation myocardial infarction; PCI, percutaneous coronary intervention; SC, subcutaneous; STEMI, ST segment elevation myocardial infarction.

be discontinued at the end of PCI, and the arterial sheath removed promptly when activated clotting time is less than 175–200.[3]

Low-Molecular-Weight Heparin

Low-molecular-weight heparin (LMWH) has a narrower spectrum of weight distribution, which renders it more predictable with respect to dose response. It has an increased half-life compared with unfractionated heparin. In addition, the incidence of heparin-induced thrombocytopenia is still present, although lower when compared with unfractionated heparin.[3] There are three commercially available LMWH, but only enoxaparin is recommended by the ACC/AHA.[3]

In the setting of non ST-segment elevation ACS, enoxaparin is administered 1 mg/kg subcutaneously every 12 hours. In the setting of ST segment elevation ACS, enoxaparin therapy is initiated with an intravenous bolus of 30 mg, followed by 1 mg/kg subcutaneous dose every 12 hours. For elderly patients (age >75), an intravenous bolus is eliminated in the setting of ST segment elevation ACS, and the maintenance dosage is reduced to 0.75 mg/kg subcutaneous every 12 hours.[3]

During PCI, an additional intravenous 0.3 mg/kg enoxaparin can be administered if the last subcutaneous dose was more than 8 hours before PCI. After PCI, the arterial sheath may be removed 6 hours after the last enoxaparin dose.[3]

Direct Thrombin Inhibitor

Bivalirudin, a synthetic peptide, is a reversible direct thrombin inhibitor. In ACS, bivalirudin therapy is initiated with a 0.1 mg/kg bolus followed by 0.25 mg/kg/hr. Just prior to PCI, an additional 0.5 mg/kg bolus followed by 1.75 mg/kg/hr is administered. If initial therapy was not administered prior to PCI, then a 0.75 mg/kg bolus, followed by 1.75 mg/kg/hr, can be administered at the time of PCI and continued up to 4 hours.[3] For creatinine clearance of less than 30 mL/min, the bivalirudin infusion rate should be reduced to 1 mg/kg/hr.

Factor Xa Inhibitor

Fondaparinux is a selective factor Xa inhibitor. Because fondaparinux therapy is associated with increased incidence of catheter-related thrombosis,[16] the guidelines recommend that fondaparinux be used in conjunction with another anticoagulant with anti–factor IIa activity during PCI.[3] Specifically, the ACC/AHA guidelines recommend an intravenous unfractionated heparin bolus (50–60 units/kg)[3].

In the setting of non–ST segment elevation ACS, a 2.5 mg subcutaneous dose is given daily. For creatinine clearance of less than 30 mL/min, fondaparinux is contraindicated.[16]

Intracoronary Vasodilators

During PCI, coronary artery vasospasm and no-reflow phenomenon can have a significant adverse impact on the procedural outcome. The following pharmacological agents can be administered intracoronary to resolve these complications (Table 2.3).

Nitrates

Nitroglycerin in various forms can be administered to provide symptom relief from angina and to control hypertension. An intracoronary nitroglycerin bolus induces vasodilatation and can resolve coronary vasospasm. Because of its antihypertensive property, the patient's blood pressure must be sufficient to tolerate nitroglycerin. A 100–200 μg intracoronary nitroglycerin bolus can be administered to improve the estimation of vessel size, as well as the severity of vessel stenosis.[17]

Table 2.3 Vasodilators and vasopressors.

| | Dosage | |
	Bolus	Infusion
Nitroglycerine	• 100–200 µg IC at a time	
Adenosine	• 100 µg IC at a time	
Calcium Channel Blockers		
Nicardipine	• Up to 200 µg IC at a time	
Diltiazem	• 1 mg IC at a time, up to 2.5 mg	
Dobutamine		• 2–20 µg per kg per minute IV
Dopamine		• 1–15 µg per kg per minute IV
Epinephrine	• 1 mg every 3–5 minutes IV	• 2–10 µg per minute IV
Phenylephrine	• 0.04–0.1 mg every 10 minutes IV	• 40–180 µg per minute IV
Norepinephrine	• 8–16 µg IV	• 0.5–30 µg per minute IV

Adenosine

Adenosine (100 µg) can be administered intracoronary for reversal of no-reflow phenomenon.[17] Because it can cause transient heart block, adenosine should be used cautiously or avoided altogether in patients with underlying heart block.

Calcium Channel Blocker

Nicardipine is a dihydropyridine calcium channel blocker that can be administered intracoronary to reverse no-reflow phenomenon. In general, boluses of up to 200 µg can be administered at a time.[17]

Diltiazem is a nondihydropyridine calcium channel blocker that can be administered intracoronary to reverse no-reflow phenomenon; 1 mg can be administered at a time and repeated up to a total of 2.5 mg.[17] Because nondihydropyridine calcium channel blockers can cause bradycardia, the patients' heart rate should be monitored closely.

Vasopressors

For the hemodynamically unstable patients presenting with ACS, vasopressor support during PCI may be critical. The following agents are readily available in catheterization laboratories around the country and should be administered promptly to improve hemodynamic status and clinical outcome (Table 2.3):

• Dobutamine is a pure β-agonist that can be administered as an intravenous infusion at 2–20 µg/kg/min.[17]

- Dopamine is a mixed α-, β-, and dopaminergic agonist that can be administered as and intravenous infusion at 1–15 μg/kg/min.[17]
- Epinephrine is a mixed α- and β-agonist that can be administered as an intravenous bolus (1 mg every 3–5 minutes) or as a continuous infusion at 2–10 μg/min.[17]
- Phenylephrine is a pure α-agonist that can be administered as an intravenous bolus (0.04–0.1 mg every 10 minutes) or as a continuous infusion at 40–180 μg/min.[17]
- Norepinephrine is a mixed α- and β-agonist that can be administered as an intravenous infusion at 0.5–30 μg/min or given as a bolus.[17]

Practical Pearls

- Antiplatelet therapy plays a key role in adjunct pharmacotherapy for PCI during elective and ACS situations.
- Prasugrel, a potent novel ADP antagonist, is contraindicated in patients with active pathological bleeding, a history of transient ischemic attacks or stroke, or in need of urgent surgery, including CABG surgery.[8]
- The ACC/AHA guidelines recommend fondaparinux use in conjunction with an intravenous unfractionated heparin bolus during PCI.[3]
- Phenylephrine, a pure α-agonist that can be administered as an intravenous bolus or as a continuous infusion, is the most commonly used vasopressor in the catheterization lab.[17]

References

1. Rosamond W, et al. Heart disease and stroke statistics—2007 update: a report from the American Heart Association Statistics Committee and Stroke Statistics Subcommittee. *Circulation*. 2007;115:e69-e171.

2. Davì G, Patrono C. Mechanisms of disease: platelet activation and atherothrombosis. *N Engl J Med*. 2007;357:2482-2494.

3. Anderson JL, et al. ACC/AHA 2007 guidelines for the management of patients with unstable angina/non–ST-elevation myocardial infarction: a report of the American College of Cardiology/American Heart Association Task Force on Practice Guidelines (Writing Committee to revise the 2002 guidelines for the management of patients with unstable angina/non–ST-elevation myocardial infarction). Developed in collaboration with the American College of Emergency Physicians, the Society for Cardiovascular Angiography and Interventions, and the Society of Thoracic Surgeons endorsed by the American Association of Cardiovascular and Pulmonary Rehabilitation and the Society for Academic Emergency Medicine. *J Am Coll Cardiol*. 2007;50:e1-e157.

4. King SB, et al. 2007 Focused Update of the ACC/AHA/SCAI 2005 Guideline Update for Percutaneous Coronary Intervention: a report of the American College of Cardiology/American Heart Association Task Force on Practice Guidelines: 2007 Writing Group to Review New Evidence and Update the ACC/AHA/SCAI 2005 Guideline Update for Percutaneous Coronary Intervention, Writing on Behalf of the 2005 Writing Committee. *Circulation*. 2008;117:261-295.

5. Yusuf S, et al. Clopidogrel in unstable angina to prevent recurrent events trial investigators. Effects of clopidogrel in addition to aspirin in patients with acute coronary syndromes without ST-segment elevation. *N Engl J Med.* 2001;345(7):494-502.

6. Antman EM, et al. 2007 Focused update of the ACC/AHA 2004 guidelines for the management of patients with ST-elevation myocardial infarction: a report of the American College of Cardiology/American Heart Association Task Force on Practice Guidelines: Developed in collaboration with the Canadian Cardiovascular Society endorsed by the American Academy of Family Physicians: 2007 Writing Group to review new evidence and update the ACC/AHA 2004 guidelines for the management of patients with ST-elevation myocardial infarction, writing on behalf of the 2004 Writing Committee. *Circulation.* 2008;117:296-329.

7. Leon MB, et al. A clinical trial comparing three antithrombotic-drug regimens after coronary-artery stenting. Stent Anticoagulation Restenosis Study Investigators. *N Engl J Med.* 1998;339(23):1665-1671.

8. Wiviott SD, TRITON-TIMI 38 Investigators, et al. Prasugrel versus clopidogrel in patients with acute coronary syndromes. *N Engl J Med.* 2007;357(20):2001-2015.

9. Wallentin L, et al. The study of Platelet Inhibition and Patient Outcomes (PLATO) investigators. Ticagrelor versus clopidogrel in patients with acute coronary syndromes. *N Engl J Med.* 2009;361.

10. Stone GW, et al. Routine upstream initiation vs deferred selective use of glyco-protein IIb/IIIa inhibitors in acute coronary syndromes. The ACUITY timing trial. *JAMA* 2009;297:591-602.

11. Giugliano RO, et al.; Early Glycoprotein IIb/IIIa Inhibition in non-ST Segment Elevation Acute Coronary Syndrome (EARLY ACS) investigators. Early versus delayed, provisional eptifibatide in acute coronary syndrome. *N Engl J Med.* 2009;360(21):2176-2190.

12. Lincoff AM, et al.; Evaluation of 7E3 for the Prevention of Ischemic Complications (EPILOG) investigators. Platelet glycoprotein IIb/IIIa receptor blockade and low dose heparin during percutaneous coronary revascularization. *N Engl J Med.* 1997;336:1689-1896.

13. Tcheng JE, et al.; Enhanced Suppression of the Platelet IIb/IIIa Receptor with Integrilin Therapy (ESPRIT) investigators. Novel dosing regimen of Eptifibatide in Planned Coronary Stent Implantation (ESPRIT): A randomized, placebo-con-trolled trial. *Lancet.* 2000;356:2037-2044.

14. Januzzi JL, et al. Benefits and safety of tirofiban among acute coronary syndrome patients with mild to moderate renal insufficiency. Results from the Platelet Receptor Inhibition in Ischemic Syndrome Management in Patients Limited by Unstable Signs and Symptoms (PRISM-PLUS) trial. *Circulation.* 2002;105:2361-2366.

15. Lee SW, et al. Triple versus dual antiplatelet therapy after coronary stenting: impact on stent thrombosis. *J Am Coll Cardiol.* 2005;46:1833-1837.

16. Yusuf S, et al.; Organization to Assess Strategies in Acute Ischemic Syndromes (OASIS) investigators. Comparison of fondaparinux and enoxaparin in acute coronary syndromes. *N Engl J Med.* 2006;354:1462-1476.

17. Baim DS, et al. *Grossman's cardiac catheterization, angiography, and intervention,* 7th ed. Philadelphia: Lippincott, Williams & Wilkins, 2006;65-71.

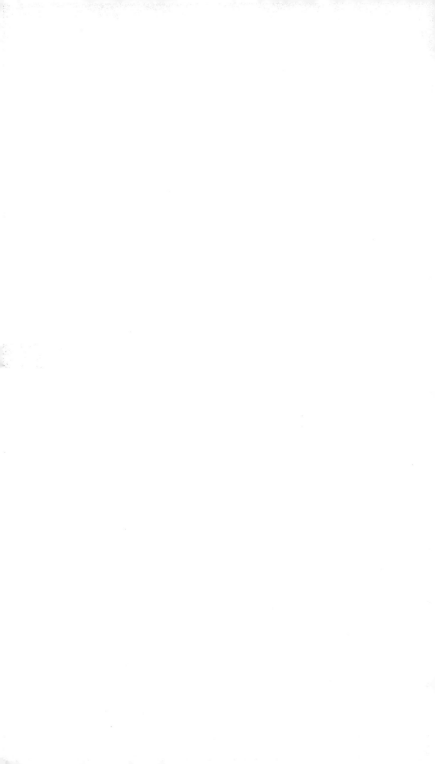

Chapter 3

Vascular Access (Femoral, Brachial, Radial): Use of Micropuncture Techniques

Rohit Bhatheja

Unarguably, vascular access has gained tremendous respect in the past few years in the modern-day cardiac catheterization laboratory. The emphasis on preventing bleeding and access complications as a major outcome or success measure of a percutaneous coronary intervention (PCI) requires careful consideration and planning, and technical precision on the part of the operator. The aim of this chapter is to describe common arterial access sites and techniques.

Arterial Access Techniques

Arterial access is usually gained through the femoral, radial, or the brachial artery. A micropuncture kit is very helpful in patients with severe peripheral arterial disease (PVD), feeble pulse, high risk of bleeding (smaller-gauge needle), and also for radial and brachial access. A 21-gauge needle (short or 7-cm long depending on the kit) is introduced into the vessel using the same technique for both femoral and radial access; then a 0.018-inch wire (stainless steel or nitinol with stainless steel or platinum tip) is advanced under fluoroscopy and placement is confirmed. A small skin incision is made, and a 4 or 5 Fr sheath/dilator assembly is introduced. This can then easily be switched to a 6, 7, or 8 Fr sheath over a 0.035–0.038-inch wire.

Some micropuncture kits, such as the Cook Micropuncture Kit (Flexor® Check-Flo®) shown in Figure 3.1, have a .018-inch nitinol wire over which the 6 Fr introducer sheath can be directly placed in the vessel without exchanging it for a 4 or 5 Fr sheath/dilator assembly. The hydrophilic coating of these sheaths, when wet, provides an extremely low coefficient of friction, thus facilitating introduction into and removal from the vascular system.

The micropuncture needle has a small lumen; hence, it may be sometimes difficult to distinguish arterial from venous blood backflow. Fluoroscopic landmarks or a small contrast injection via the 4 Fr sheath helps identify the vessel.

The Bard Micropuncture Kit (Fig. 3.2) has a radiopaque sheath, making it easily visualized. A micropuncture kit is a must for laboratories doing peripheral vascular cases.

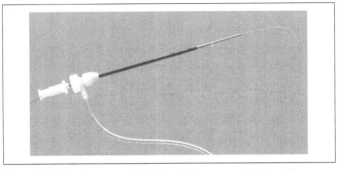

Figure 3.1 Cook micropuncture kit. This radial artery access kit utilizes a 21-gauge needle for arterial access, over which a 0.018-inch nitinol wire is advanced. The outer surface of the introducer and the distal tip of the inner dilator are coated with AQ® hydrophilic coating. Depending on the manufacturer, sheaths are available in long (23 cm), standard (13 cm), and short (7 cm) lengths.

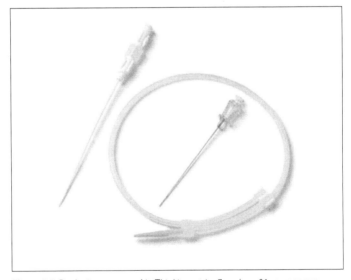

Figure 3.2 Bard micropuncture kit. This kit contains 7-cm-long, 21-gauge access needle with echogenic tip, a 45-cm-long, 0.018-inch guidewire, stainless steel or nitinol, with stainless steel or platinum tips and a locking 10-cm sheath/dilator assembly. The radiopaque sheath, dilator, and needle are easily visualized.

Femoral Arterial Access

Which Side?

The right groin is accessed more frequently than the left because the operator is on the right side of the patient. This reduces inadvertent loss of access during manipulation of the manifold. However, patient preference, anatomic reasons (presence of hernia or infected/indurated groin area), and previous scars and surgeries—especially bypass grafts—are important considerations to keep in mind when selecting the appropriate groin site.

Technique

Arterial access for coronary catheterization is most commonly gained via retrograde common femoral arterial (CFA) puncture using Seldinger's technique and utilizing an anterior wall stick of the CFA. The femoral artery is large enough to accommodate both large-sized sheaths for complex coronary and valvular interventions and also a balloon pump. The skin and the periadventitia over the point of entry into the femoral artery are anesthetized with lidocaine. The femoral artery is entered with a Cook needle about 1 cm below the inguinal ligament till a flash of blood is obtained, then a guidewire is introduced. A small skin incision is made (just big enough for the sheath to enter the skin site), and the wire and the dilator are removed. The sheath is attached to the manifold, flushed, and good pressure waveform is confirmed.

The femoral artery traverses the medial third of the femoral head in 97% of patients.[1] Fluoroscopy is recommended at all times to delineate the entry site,

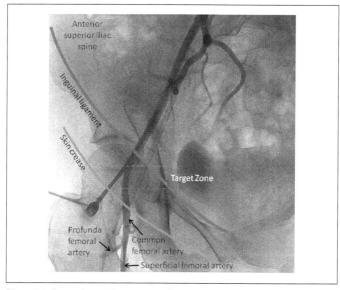

Figure 3.3 Femoral arterial access using fluoroscopic landmarks.

which should be above the bifurcation of the common femoral artery but below the origin of the inferior epigastric artery. This corresponds to the middle third of the medial edge of the femoral head on fluoroscopy (Fig. 3.3). It is important to understand that the skin entry site should be 1–2 cm lower (depending on body habitus) than the skin marking corresponding with the middle of the femoral head. This is because the needle is entered at approximately a 60-degree angle to the skin; by the time the needle traverses the skin and subcutaneous tissue, it is already directed cephalad. Meticulous attention to this detail will avoid high-entry sticks to the femoral artery. This is important in both obese and lean patients, and retraction of the pannus with the help of tape is important in obese patients to keep the tissue layer over the arteriotomy site thin and taut.

A higher arteriotomy increases the risk for retroperitoneal bleeds, whereas too low a cannulation predisposes to superficial femoral artery cannulation and its attendant risks of dissection, pseudoaneurysms, and arteriovenous fistula formation.

Although a micropuncture kit is not routinely used, in patients with large pannus or severe PVD it may be helpful in decreasing the complication rate. Absence of a groin pulse due to PVD may necessitate either ultrasound or Doppler-guided access (Smart Needle), or even switching to radial access. Directly accessing the brachial artery with a good palpable pulse, in the setting of an acute coronary syndrome requiring quick access with feeble or absent femoral pulses, may save time and myocardium (personal experience).

Complications related to femoral artery access include:

- Hematoma (1%–3%)
- Retroperitoneal hematoma (0.2%–0.9%)
- Arterial venous fistula (<0.5%)
- Pseudoaneurysms (1%–6%)
- Acute limb ischemia/acute arterial thrombosis (<0.1%):
  - Dissection, distal embolization, small vessel
  - Use of closure device (suture, collagen plug)

Practical Pearls

- Fluoroscopically guided access and proper deployment of the closure device will prevent the majority of complications.
- Always examine all pulses (radial, brachial, and femoral) before draping the patient.
- If the patient has no palpable femoral pulse, use fluoroscopic landmarks, arterial calcification, or Doppler needle (SmartNeedle) or switch to radial access (author's preference). Begin with micropuncture kit.
- If you get vein first: leave the wire in and immediately go slightly lateral to this wire to access the artery and insert the sheath. Remove the venous wire and hold pressure for 2–5 minutes.
- In cases of inability to advance a sheath, advance the wire more; avoid advancing the sheath over the floppy part of the wire. Sometimes predilation with a 5 Fr dilator or exchanging for a stiffer wire over a 4 Fr catheter may be required. *Never push the wire against resistance.* Rotational torque is the key.

- Access via bypass graft in the groin is possible if the graft is at least 4 weeks old. Access should be at an angle of 30 to 45 degrees to avoid kinking of the catheter. Puncture should be made proximal to the anastomosis site (usually proximal to the inguinal incision).
- Longer sheath lengths are useful in patients with PVD and aortic aneurysms (avoiding long catheter exchanges) and in obese patients.

Transradial Access

Compared to femoral access, transradial artery (TRA) access is safer, easier, has lower procedure costs, leads to earlier patient mobilization, and is associated with fewer bleeding complications and a corresponding trend for reduction in ischemic events. Routine use of a micropuncture kit or a dedicated radial artery access set with a hydrophilic sheath is associated with most success.

Ulno-Palmar Arch Assessment

The following tests may be done to assess the adequacy of collateral circulation to the radial artery:

- *Modified Allen's Test (MAT):* The hand is held in a supine position and the radial and ulnar arteries are compressed simultaneously. The patient is asked to clench the hand several times, causing blanching of the palm. The compression of the ulnar artery is then released and the time to achieve maximal palmar blush is noted: normal is <5 seconds, abnormal is >10 seconds, anything in between is intermediate.
- *Plethysmography (PL) and pulse oximetry (OX) (Barbeau Index)* (Fig. 3.4): Place the detector on the thumb and compress the radial artery. Measure PL and OX at 2 minutes.[2]
- *Doppler ultrasound* can be used for direct assessment of palmar circulation.

Abnormal MAT, PL, and OX tests should prompt the operator to seek an alternate access site.

Although the choice of access side is operator dependent, left-sided radial artery access facilitates coronary and left internal mammary graft cannulation. Left-sided access may be associated with less stroke risk due to the separate origin of the left internal carotid and may be preferable to right-handed patients.

Arterial Puncture and Sheath Selection

The wrist area is slightly hyperextended, and access is obtained with micropuncture or a 19-gauge needle in the straight portion of the radial artery that is 2 cm proximal to the styloid process (Fig. 3.5). Immediately after sheath insertion, a spasmolytic cocktail consisting of 2.5–5 mg of verapamil and 200 µg of nitroglycerine is administered intra-arterially. To prevent the potentially lethal complication of radial artery occlusion, anticoagulation is achieved by injecting 3,000–5,000 units of intra-arterial heparin. Approximately 10% of patients may develop radial artery spasm. The use of hydrophilic-coated sheaths is associated with less arterial spasm during sheath removal. Confirmation of good pressure

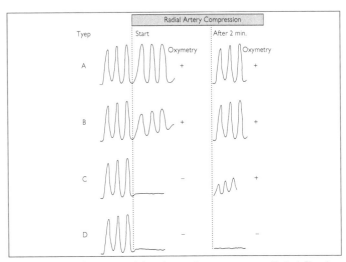

Figure 3.4 Four different types of ulnopalmar arch patency as assessed by both PL and OX with transducer applied on the thumb: (a) no dampening, (b) slight dampening of pressure tracing, (c) loss followed by recovery, (d) no recovery within 2 minutes. OX positive: oximetry present and constant; OX negative: no reading during compression. Reprinted from Barbeau GR, Arsenault F, Dugas L, Simard S, Lariviere MM. Evaluation of the ulnopalmar arterial arches with pulse oximetry and plethysmography: Comparison with the Allen's test in 1010 patients. *Am Heart J* 2004;147:489-493, with permission of the publisher (Elsevier).

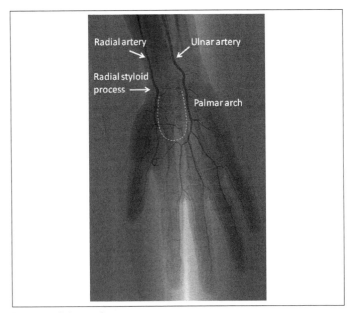

Figure 3.5 Palmar arch.

waveform and advancement of the 0.035-inch wire under fluoroscopy into the ascending aorta is done, then the diagnostic catheter is advanced over this wire. Catheters are now available that can engage both left and right coronary arteries, thus obviating the need for catheter exchanges, which is typically done over an exchange-length (260-cm) J-tipped 0.035-inch wire.

Anatomical variation in the normal radial artery (Fig. 3.6) may be encountered in up to 14% of cases, with a similar 14% rate of procedural failure. Anomalies include high bifurcating radial artery (above the intercondylar line of humerus) (Fig. 3.7), full radial loop (Fig. 3.8), extreme tortuosity, accessory branches, and radial atherosclerosis.[3] It is extremely important to remove the sheath meticulously after the procedure is over. Hemostasis can be achieved with specifically tailored radial compression systems (TR Band; Terumo Medical, Tokyo, Japan, or RADI-Stop; Radi Medical Systems, Uppsala, Sweden) (Fig. 3.9).

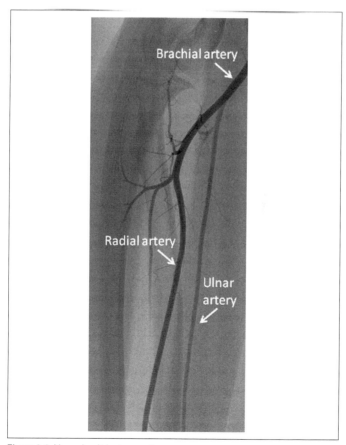

Figure 3.6 Normal radial artery anatomy.

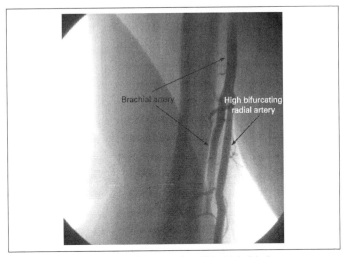

Figure 3.7 High bifurcating radial artery at the middle third of the humerus.
Reprinted from Lo TS, Nolan J, Fountzopoulos E, et al. Radial artery anomaly and its
influence on transradial coronary procedural outcome. *Heart.* 2009;95:410-415, with
permission of the publisher (Elsevier).

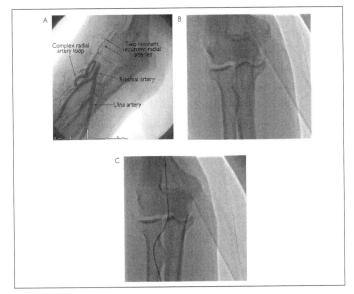

Figure 3.8 Radial artery intervention. (A) Radial artery loop; (B) crossing and straight-
ening the loop with a 0.014-inch guidewire and then inserting a 4F catheter (C) with a
counterclockwise rotation. Reprinted from Lo TS, Nolan J, Fountzopoulos E, et al. Radial
artery anomaly and its influence on transradial coronary procedural outcome. *Heart.*
2009;95:410-415, with permission of the publisher (Elsevier).

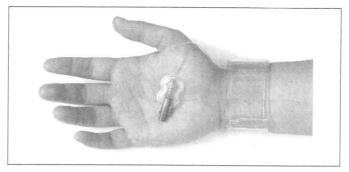

Figure 3.9 TR Band radial compression system.

Complications Related to Radial Artery Access

- Hematoma, bleeding, pseudoaneurysms, arterial thrombosis/occlusion, dissection (1%–2%)
- Stroke/brain emb olization during manipulation of the right subclavian (1%–2%)

Practical Pearls

- It is mandatory to do ulno-palmar arch assessment before radial artery access.
- Slight hyperextension of the wrist, minimal infiltration of lidocaine, and single stick of the artery just proximal to the wrist crease are keys to success.
- Always secure the sheath with sterile dressing or a silk suture.
- Use hydrophilic sheaths.
- Prep the groin (if anticipating balloon pump, severe subclavian disease).
- Always advance the wire under fluoroscopy.
- Recognize the anatomical variations of the radial artery.
- Transradial artery access is preferred over brachial.
- Remove the sheath promptly post procedure.

Brachial Artery

A brachial artery approach is usually reserved for patients with (a) inadequate ulno-palmar collaterals precluding TRA, or (b) cases in which femoral access cannot be done due to severe PVD, and (c) when larger sheaths (7-F or more) are needed and cannot be used via TRA.[4] Also, in situations involving lower extremity interventions, this approach provides a longer working length than TRA.

Technique

The area over the antecubital fossa is prepped and draped, and the arm is placed in supination with slight abduction. After local anesthesia, using a

21-gauge needle, percutaneous access to the brachial artery is obtained just proximal to the skin fold, medial to the biceps tendon (Fig. 3.10). The sheath is then inserted and stabilized either with a dressing or a suture.

Complications

- Dissection, thrombotic occlusion, hematoma formation, pseudoaneurysm, median nerve compression
- Risk is higher with operators who use this technique infrequently.

Practical Pearls

- Try to use TRA instead of brachial access unless there is a need for larger sheaths (7-F or more), lower extremity interventions, or abnormal Allen's test.
- Prompt sheath removal post-procedure, use of arm board, and frequent pulse/limb check are critical to minimize complications.
- Transradial artery or brachial access is contraindicated in patients with Buerger disease, Raynaud disease, and known upper extremity vascular disease.

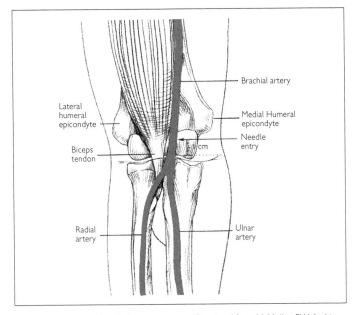

Figure 3.10 Normal brachial artery anatomy. Reprinted from McMullen PW, Jenkins JS. Arterial access for endovascular interventions: radial and brachial arterial access. In: Heuser RR, Henry M, eds. *Textbook of peripheral vascular interventions.* Informa HealthCare; 2008:21-25, with permission of the publisher.

References

1. Grier D, Hartnell G. Percutaneous femoral artery puncture: practice and anatomy. *Br J Radiol.* 1990;63:602-604.

2. Barbeau GR, Arsenault F, Dugas L, Simard S, Lariviere MM. Evaluation of the ulnopalmar arterial arches with pulse oximetry and plethysmography: comparison with the Allen's test in 1010 patients. *Am Heart J.* 2004;147:489-493.

3. Lo TS, Nolan J, Fountzopoulos E, et al. Radial artery anomaly and its influence on transradial coronary procedural outcome. *Heart.* 2009;95:410-415.

4. McMullen PW, Jenkins JS. Arterial access for endovascular interventions: radial and brachial arterial access. In: Heuser RR, Henry M, eds., *Textbook of peripheral vascular interventions.* New York: Informa HealthCare, 2008;21-25.

Chapter 4

Guiding Catheters, Guidewires, Balloon Catheters, and Cutting Balloons

Arijit Dasgupta and Sharat Koul

The most important step in the safe and successful performance of percutaneous coronary intervention (PCI) remains the operator's ability to select the appropriate guiding catheter, guidewire, and balloon catheter for each case.[1] This chapter reviews the design of these pieces of interventional equipment and the steps to consider in their selection.

Guiding Catheters

The role of the guiding catheter in PCI is summarized in Table 4.1.

To accomplish all of these objectives, the operator should address the following questions prior to catheter selection (Table 4.2).

Support

Table 4.3 summarizes the concept of support.

As seen in Table 4.3, passive support is a function of the guiding catheter and aortic root factors. These factors are summarized in Table 4.4.

Table 4.1 Guiding catheter objectives

Provide adequate support for the specific PCI procedure to be performed.
Provide safe, coaxial engagement to the specific coronary ostium.
Allow injection of contrast and passage of interventional equipment through the coronary artery.

Table 4.2 Questions to address prior to guiding catheter selection

How much support is needed for the specific PCI?
What is the target coronary artery take-off anatomy?
What is the guiding catheter luminal size needed?

Support	
	Ability of a guiding catheter to accommodate forward passage of interventional equipment through the coronary vasculature without prolapse of its tip back into the aorta/aortic sinus[1]
Types of Support	*Passive support*: provided by properties of the guide catheter and its interaction with the aortic root
	Active support: provided by operator-dependent techniques (e.g., deep-seating the guide into the coronary artery)

Table 4.4 Factors affecting the passive support of a guide catheter

Increased Passive Support Provided	Decreased Passive Support Provided
Larger luminal diameter (7 Fr, 8 Fr, 9 Fr)	Smaller luminal diameter (6 Fr, 5 Fr)
Larger angle between catheter secondary curve and contralateral aortic wall	Smaller angle between catheter secondary curve and contralateral aortic wall
Longer length of contact between catheter secondary curve and contralateral aortic wall	Shorter length of contact between catheter secondary curve and contralateral aortic wall
Inherent stiffness of catheter due to wire braid/nylon construction	Lack of wire braid/nylon in catheter construction

Figure 4.1 illustrates the importance of the interaction of the aortic wall with the guiding catheter in enhancing passive support[2].

Guiding catheter construction is a key component of support.[3] Figure 4.2 illustrates the composite three-layer design found in modern guiding catheters: an inner lining of Teflon or polytetrafluoroethylene (PTFE) affords a low coefficient of friction to allow smooth balloon and/or stent passage, a middle layer of fine braided wire provides stiffness and torque control capability, and an outer layer of nylon blends increases the strength of the catheter. Most catheters also have a smooth exterior coating, which is nonthrombogenic.

Figure 4.3 summarizes clinical scenarios in which differing amounts of support are needed.

Coaxial Engagement

Due to significant variations in the take-off of the coronary arteries from the aortic cusps, coaxial engagement is often not straightforward. The typical orientation of the left main coronary artery (LMCA) is an orthogonal projection from the middle portion of the anterior left coronary sinus just inferior to the sinotubular junction.[4] Figure 4.4 demonstrates variant LMCA take-off. Similarly, the typical right coronary artery (RCA) orientation is an orthogonal projection from the middle of the right anterior coronary sinus just inferior to the sinotubular junction.[4] There is considerably more variation of the RCA ostium in terms of location in the sinus and orientation of take-off compared to the LMCA. Figure 4.5 illustrates the most common variants of the RCA ostium. Figure 4.6 summarizes some appropriate guides that can be used to cannulate

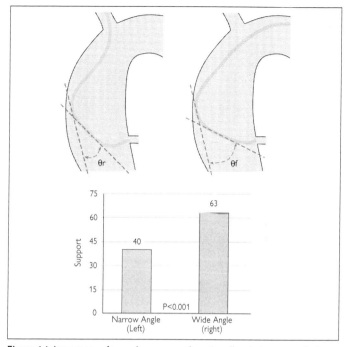

Figure 4.1 Importance of secondary curve and aortic wall angle in support. Ikari et al.[2] performed elegant experiments to analyze the physics of support provided by guiding catheters. Their findings confirmed the clinical experience that support is affected by two aortic root factors: (1) the angle the catheter makes with the contralateral aortic wall, and (2) the length of the contact area of the catheter against the contralateral wall. This highlights the importance of considering aortic root dimensions in determining the likely amount of support provided by the guiding catheter. θ refers to angle between catheter and contralateral wall; r, radial access; f, femoral access. Reprinted from Ikari Y, Nagaoka M, Kim JY, Morino Y, Tanabe T. The physics of guiding catheters for the left coronary artery in transfemoral and transradial interventions. *J Invas Cardiol.* 2005;17:636-641, with permission of the publisher (HMP Communications).

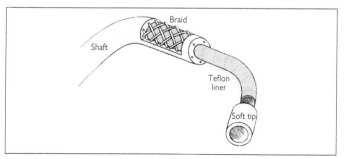

Figure 4.2 Features of guide catheters. Reprinted from Holmes DR, Mathew V. *Atlas of interventional cardiology*, 2nd ed. Philadelphia: Current Medicine, Inc.; 2003, with permission of the publisher (Current Medicine Group LLC).

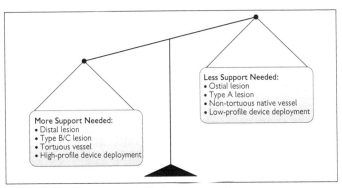

Figure 4.3 Clinical scenarios with differing support needs.

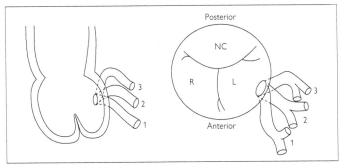

Figure 4.4 Variations in left coronary artery (LMCA) take-off. The projection of the LMCA can vary in terms of both a superior/inferior plane (*left*) and an anterior/posterior plane (*right*). Frontal and horizontal views showing the three most common variations of the origin of the left coronary artery. On the left figure, 1, inferior tilt; 2, normal orthogonal origin; and 3, superior tilt. For the figure on the right, 1, anterior tilt; 2, normal orthogonal origin; and 3, posterior tilt. NC, Noncoronary sinus; R, right coronary sinus; L, left coronary sinus. Reprinted from Ellis SG, Holmes DR. *Strategic approaches in coronary intervention*, 3rd ed. Philadelphia: Lippincott Williams & Wilkins, 2006, with permission of the publisher (Wolters Kluwer Health).

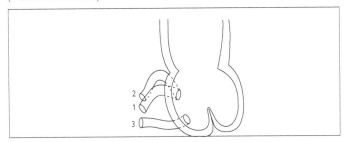

Figure 4.5 Variations in right coronary artery (RCA) take-off. The most common variants of RCA origin variation are (1) normal, (2) shepherd's crook, and (3) low ectopic origin with horizontal course. Reprinted from Ellis SG, Holmes DR. *Strategic approaches in coronary intervention*, 3rd ed. Philadelphia: Lippincott Williams & Wilkins, 2006, with permission of the publisher (Wolters Kluwer Health).

these types of variant coronary take-offs[5] (e.g., anterior, posterior, inferior, superior, and high take-offs) but, in the majority of cases, clinical trial and error will dictate the most appropriate guide.

Guide Lumen Size

Currently, the guiding catheter size for routine PCI is 6 Fr, although some operators are starting to use 5 Fr systems for standard cases. The 7 or 8 Fr catheters are commonly used in cases with bifurcation lesions or complex coronary anatomy requiring rotablation.

Typical Guides

In the modern era, guiding catheters are available in all conventional Judkins (left and right) and Amplatz (left and right) shapes, as well as in a wide range of custom shapes, for example, extra back-up (XB) and multipurpose (MPA). All shapes come with a soft, radiopaque tip to minimize ostial trauma on engagement (Fig. 4.7).

The key features of these common guiding catheters and their associated advantages and disadvantages are summarized in Table 4.5.

Figure 4.8 illustrates the properly sized Judkins Left (JL) catheter compared to an oversized and undersized JL catheter.

Amplatz guides are especially useful for PCI involving the left circumflex[6] (LCX), as the Judkins left tends to point toward the left anterior descending

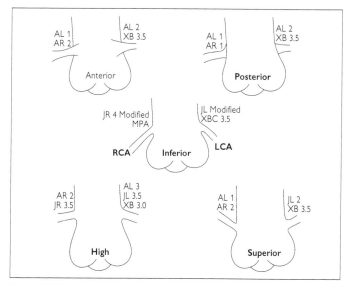

Figure 4.6 Coronary variations and appropriate guide catheters. From Cordis Corporation. *Cordis VistaBrite Tip; Shapes for variable take-offs.* Johnson & Johnson, 2007, with permission of the publisher.

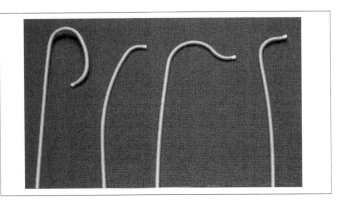

Figure 4.7 Commonly used angioplasty guide catheters for the native coronary arteries. From left to right, the Judkins left (JL) coronary curve, the Judkins right (JR) curve, the Amplatz left (AL) coronary curve, and the Amplatz right (AR) coronary curve. Reprinted from Holmes DR, Mathew V. *Atlas of interventional cardiology*, 2nd ed. Philadelphia: Current Medicine, Inc., 2003, with permission of the publisher (Current Medicine Group LLC).

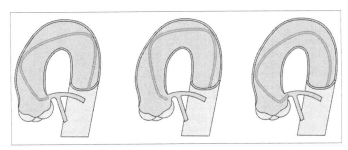

Figure 4.8 Judkins catheter position. The appropriate size of a JL guide catheter is based on the width of the patient's ascending aorta. *Left:* The properly sized JL guide easily engages the left coronary ostium as the tip tends to automatically move upward and find the left coronary ostium once the guidewire is removed. If it does not, once in the left coronary sinus, gentle counterclockwise rotation will direct the guide anteriorly where it will usually find the left main coronary artery ostium. *Middle:* A JL guide that remains in the vertical axis of the ascending aorta and whose tip points down in the aortic sinus is too large and should be changed for a smaller size. *Right:* A JL guide that has either refolded in the aortic root or whose tip points up is too small and should be changed for a larger size. Reprinted from Holmes DR, Mathew V. *Atlas of interventional cardiology*, 2nd ed. Philadelphia: Current Medicine, Inc., 2003, with permission of the publisher (Current Medicine Group LLC).

Table 4.5 Features of common guiding catheters

Name	Curvature	Size (cm)	Advantages	Disadvantages
Judkins Left (JL)	1° curve: 90 degrees 2° curve: 180 degrees	Determined by length of arm between 1° and 2° curves: JL3.5, JL4, JL5, JL6	• Adequate for straightforward LAD PCI cases • May be best choice in ostial lesions	• Sharp primary curve may limit coaxial alignment in many cases • Poor support in complex LCX cases
Judkins Right (JR)	1° curve: 90 degrees 2° curve:30 degrees	Determined by length of secondary curve: JR3.5, JR4, JR5, JR6	• Adequate for simple RCA PCI cases	Primary curve limits coaxial engagement in anterior RCA and superiorly RCA take-off
Amplatz Right (AR)	1° curve: tapered tip perpendicular to secondary curve 2° curve: pre-shaped half circle	Determined by length of secondary curve: AL1-AL3, AR1-AR3	• Provides excellent support for most complex PCI • Appropriate for LCX lesion • Useful in cases where JL/JR guides unable to provide adequate support	May not be useful and is not recommended for ostial lesions
Extra Back-Up (XB)	Straight tip with long circular curve	Determined by length of secondary curve: XB3.0, XB 3.5, XB4.0	• Provides excellent support due to long circular curve laying against contralateral aortic wall • Commonly used in most labs as workforce guide for left coronary interventions	May not be appropriate for very short left main
Multipurpose (MPA)	Straight with single minor bend at tip (primary curve)		Can be used for hard to engage grafts	Not used commonly

PCI, percutaneous coronary intervention; LAD, left anterior descending; LCX, left circumflex; RCA, right coronary artery.

(LAD) artery, and also for the RCA with an anterior or superior take-off. The appropriate positioning of an Amplatz guide is illustrated in Figure 4.9.

The XB catheter is an excellent guide catheter used predominantly in complex LAD/LCX lesions. Figure 4.10 summarizes its appropriate positioning.

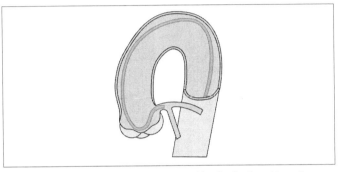

Figure 4.9 **Appropriate left Amplatz guide position.** Use of an Amplatz guide requires proper sizing of the aortic root. The smallest root requires an AL1, a normal root in a male requires an AL2 (usually a smaller size is required for women), and a large aortic root needs an AL3. If the tip of the Amplatz does not reach the ostium and lies below it, the guide is too small; conversely, if the tip lies above the ostium it is too large. Engagement of the left main coronary artery is achieved by counterclockwise rotation and advancement in the right anterior oblique projection. The secondary curve usually lies in the noncoronary cusp when engaging the left main coronary. Withdrawal of the guide requires further advancement until the tip prolapses out of the ostium, followed by rotation. Simply withdrawing the catheter risks further deep seating and possible ostial trauma. Reprinted from Douglas JS. Selection and use of basic equipment, guiding catheters, wires, and balloons. In: Kern MJ, Berger PB, Block PC, Klein L, Laskey W, eds. *SCAI Interventional Cardiology Board review book.* Philadelphia: Lippincott Williams & Wilkins, 2006, with permission of the publisher (Wolters Kluwer Health).

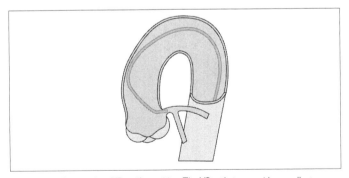

Figure 4.10 **Appropriate XB guide position.** The XB catheter provides excellent support for complex PCI cases due to its long curve resting against the contralateral aortic wall. Engagement of the left main coronary artery by this catheter is usually straightforward and relies on clockwise and counterclockwise rotation in the RAO projection. Reprinted from Douglas JS. Selection and use of basic equipment, guiding catheters, wires, and balloons. In: Kern MJ, Berger PB, Block PC, Klein L, Laskey W, eds. *SCAI Interventional Cardiology Board review book.* Philadelphia: Lippincott Williams & Wilkins, 2006, with permission of the publisher (Wolters Kluwer Health).

Algorithms for Guide Selection

Figures 4.11–4.13 summarize general algorithms for guide catheter selection, based on clinical practice.

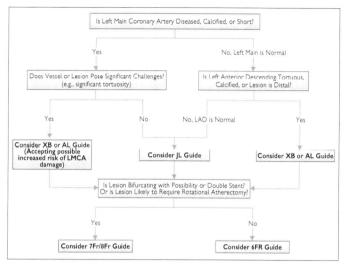

Figure 4.11 Guide selection algorithm for left anterior descending (LAD)-based interventions. (Note: algorithm assumes femoral arterial access is applicable to most clinical scenarios, but may not apply in anomalous or variant coronary artery take-offs.)

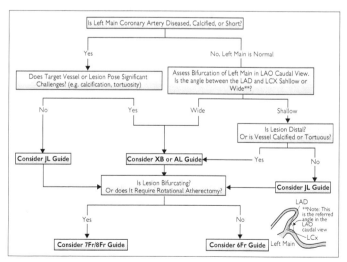

Figure 4.12 Guide selection algorithm for left circumflex (LCX)-based interventions. (Note: algorithm assumes femoral arterial access and is applicable to most clinical scenarios, but it may not apply in anomalous or variant coronary artery take-offs.)

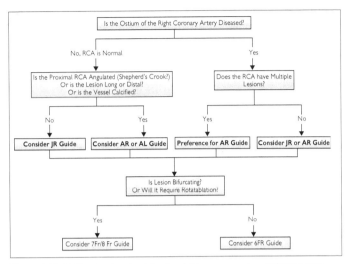

Figure 4.13 Guide selection algorithm for right coronary artery (RCA) interventions. (Note: algorithm assumes femoral arterial access is applicable to most clinical scenarios, but may not apply in anomalous or variant coronary artery take-offs.)

Table 4.6 Guidewire design

Design Element	Composition
Central core	Stainless steel or nitinol; usually 145 cm long
Distal tip	Core taper with polymer sleeve vs. wire coil spring; usually distal 20–40 cm
Coating	Hydrophobic or hydrophilic

Guidewires

The modern guidewire has three main components[4] (Table 4.6 and Fig. 4.14).

The differing characteristics of guidewires are due to variations in the listed components, and they can be described in terms of six main features, as shown in Table 4.7.[7]

The design of the distal tip in terms of central core taper and weld design plays a major role in determining the property of the wire. Overall, there is a tradeoff between torquability, support, malleability, and trackability on one side and flexibility on the other. Figure 4.15 illustrates the effect of core taper on wire properties, and Figure 4.16 illustrates the effect of tip weld design on wire property.

The final step in the construction of a guidewire includes radiopacity provided by platinum coils and the application of an outer coating, which can be either hydrophobic, hydrophilic, or a hybrid.

Table 4.7 Guidewire features

Feature	Definition	Design Component
Stiffness	Strength of wire	Core composition, core diameter, and length of core taper; stainless steel, large diameter, and short taper with increased strength
Flexibility	Ability of wire to bend with direct pressure; relates to wire's ability to cross lesions without causing endothelial trauma	Core composition, core diameter, length of core taper, tip design; nitinol, smaller diameter, longer core taper, and shaping ribbon tip with increased flexibility
Torquability	Ability of wire to transmit rotational forces from proximal to distal tip; relates to wire's ability to advance through tortuous vessels	Core composition, core diameter, length/type of core taper, and tip design; stainless steel, large diameter, short taper with parabolic taper, and core-to-tip design with increased torquability
Malleability	Ability of wire to attain and retain desired shape	Tip design; shaping ribbon tip increases malleability
Trackability	Ability of wire body to follow tortuous course and ability of balloon to trail along guidewire	Core composition, core diameter, and length of core taper; stainless steel, large diameter, and short taper with increased trackability
Tactile feedback	Feel of wire tip behavior as perceived by operator	Coating; hydrophilic coat decreases tactile feedback

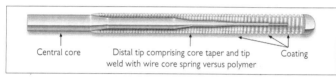

Central core   Distal tip comprising core taper and tip weld with wire core spring versus polymer   Coating

Figure 4.14 Wire construction.

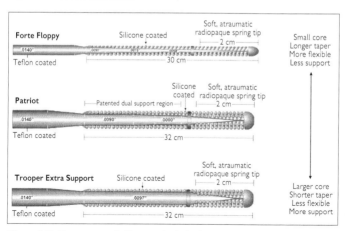

Figure 4.15 Core taper and effect on wire behavior.

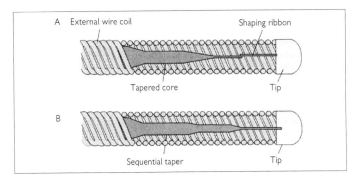

Figure 4.16 Guidewire tip design. At the distal segment of the wire, where the core starts to taper, stainless steel coils can cover the tip and tapered core. A variation is the use of a proprietary polymer coat in the distal portion instead of stainless steel coils. The effect of these coils or polymer coats is to keep the diameter of the wire constant as the core tapers and also to add flexibility to the distal portion of the wire. Wires can be constructed either with (A) the core attached to the tip weld via a shaping ribbon (shaping ribbon construction) or (B) the core extending all the way to the tip with the core being flattened at the tip (uniweld/core-to-tip construction). The shaping ribbon construction produces a floppy tip with increased flexibility but decreased torquability, whereas the uniweld design give increased tip control but decreased flexibility. Reprinted from Holmes DR, Mathew V. *Atlas of interventional cardiology*, 2nd ed. Philadelphia: Current Medicine, Inc., 2003, with permission of the publisher (Current Medicine Group LLC).

Table 4.8 Guidewire selection issues

PCI Scenario	Wire Requirements
Regular coronary anatomy	Moderate flexibility, moderate support
Tortuous coronary anatomy	Torquability and trackability properties become most important
High support requirements	Support is most important
Chronic total occlusion (CTO)	Support, torquability important; usually with uniweld tip design, short core taper, hydrophilic coating

Guidewire Selection

Guidewire selection is based on the specific PCI scenario and can be classified into four general groups,[5] as summarized in Table 4.8.

The best approach to guidewire choice is to select a "workhorse" wire for each of the scenarios summarized in Table 4.8 and become thoroughly familiar with the selected wire's behavior. Once workhorse wire behavior is mastered, the operator can expand to other wires if the workhorse wire is unlikely to be adequate for a certain clinical scenario. Table 4.9 summarizes some appropriate workhorse wire choices for each of these clinical scenarios.

Table 4.9 Workhorse wires

Regular Anatomy	Tortuous Anatomy	Extra Support	CTO
Balance Middle Weight (BMW)/BMW Universal (Abbott)	Whisper wire (Abbott)	Balance Heavyweight (Boston Scientific/ Guidant)	Asahi Miracle Bros (Abbott)
Asahi Light (Abbott)	CholCE PT Floppy (Boston Scientific/ Guidant)	Ironman (Boston Scientific/Guidant)	Confianza (Abbott)
CholCE Floppy (Boston Scientific/ Guidant)	Asahi Prowater (Abbott)	CholCE Extra support (Boston Scientific/Guidant)	Cross-IT (Boston Scientific/ Guidant)
High Torque Floppy (Boston Scientific/ Guidant)	PT Graphix (Boston Scientific/Guidant)	Mailman (Boston Scientific/Guidant)	Pilot (Abbott)
CTO, chronic total occlusion.			

Table 4.10 summarizes the specifications of common workhorse guidewires.

Guidewire Handling

Once the appropriate wire has been selected, the operator should shape a curve at its distal tip to help guide entry into the artery of interest:

• A large, broad curve will select the LAD over the LCX.

• A sharper curve will select the LCX or branch vessel.

Once the wire is in the artery of interest, it must be advanced through the lesion into the distal coronary vasculature. This is accomplished through a combination of torquing and steering of the selected wire. Although all operators have differing specific technical preferences regarding the appropriate combination of steering with torquing of the wire, most operators use their right hand to manipulate a torquing device by 180 degrees via repetitive clockwise/counterclockwise rotation, while their left hand is used to steer and advance the wire. As the wire is being advanced, the operator must constantly observe the wire to ensure the tip does not prolapse. If prolapse occurs, it suggests that the tip is catching on an atherosclerotic lesion, and further advancement risks intimal injury. The wire should be promptly withdrawn until the prolapse reverts, then rotate the tip and advance the wire again. This technique is repeated until the wire safely reaches the distal vasculature. Following this, the appropriate balloon catheter is selected and advanced over the wire.

Table 4.10 Specifications of common workhorse guidewires

Wire Type (Manufacturer)	Support	Core Material	Tip Flexibility	Tip Style	Tip Design	Coating
Regular Anatomy Wires (0.014")						
Choice Floppy (Boston Scientific)	Light	Stainless steel	Floppy	Springcoil	Uniweld	Hydrophilic with distal tip uncoated
Whisper (Abbott)	Light/Moderate	Stainless steel	Intermediate	Polymer	Uniweld	Hydrophilic
BMW (Abbott)	Moderate	Stainless steel/ Nitinol composite	Floppy	Springcoil	Shaping ribbon	Hydrophilic with distal tip uncoated
Asahi Light (Abbott)	Light/Moderate	Stainless steel	Floppy	Springcoil	Uniweld	Hydrophobic
Reflex (Cordis)	Light	Stainless steel	Floppy	Platinum coil	Uniweld	Hydrophobic
Tortuous Anatomy Wires (0.014")						
Choice PT Floppy (Boston Scientific)	Light	Stainless steel	Intermediate	Polymer	Uniweld	Hydrophilic
PT2 Light (Boston Scientific)	Light	Nitinol	Intermediate	Polymer	Shaping ribbon	Hydrophilic
Whisper (Abbott)	Light/Moderate	Stainless steel	Intermediate	Polymer	Uniweld	Hydrophilic
Asahi Prowater (Abbott)	Moderate	Stainless steel	Intermediate	Springcoil	Uniweld	Hybrid distal hydrophobic/ proximal hydrophilic

PT Graphix (Boston Scientific)	Moderate	Stainless steel	Intermediate	Polymer	Uniweld	Hydrophilic
PT2 Moderate (Boston Scientific)	Moderate	Nitinol	Intermediate	Polymer	Shaping ribbon	Hydrophilic
Heavy Support Wires (0.014")						
Choice PT Extrasupport (Boston Scientific)	Extra	Stainless steel	Intermediate	Polymer	Uniweld	Hydrophilic
Mailman (Boston Scientific)	Super	Stainless steel	Floppy	Springcoil	Uniweld	Hydrophilic with distal tip uncoated
Stabilizer Plus (Cordis)	Heavy/Extra Support	Stainless steel	Floppy	Springcoil	Uniweld	Hydrophilic with distal tip uncoated
Chronic Total Occlusion (0.014")						
Miracle Bros 3, 4.5, 6, 12 (Abbott)	Moderate, Extra, Super	Stainless steel	Intermediate/Stiff	Springcoil	Uniweld	Hydrophilic
Confianza (Abbott)	Extra/Super	Stainless steel	Stiff	Springcoil	Uniweld	Hydrophobic
Cross-IT (Abbott)	Moderate	Stainless steel	Intermediate/Stiff	Springcoil/ Polymer fusion	Uniweld	Hydrophilic
Other (0.009")						
RotaWire (Boston Scientific)	Light	Stainless steel	Floppy	N/A	N/A	N/A

Table 4.11 Balloon properties

Property	Definition
Compliance	Change in balloon diameter as a function of inflation pressure; clinically refers to the strength of radial force direction of an inflated balloon
Profile	Maximum diameter of the deflated balloon when mounted on a catheter; clinically refers to the diameter the deflated balloon can pass through
Nominal	Pressure at which the balloon reaches its package label diameter
Rated burst pressure	Pressure threshold at which in vitro testing has shown 99.9% of the specified balloons will not burst
Mean burst pressure	Average pressure at which the specified balloon will burst

Balloon Catheters

Table 4.11 defines the important properties of the balloon mounted on the balloon catheter.[8] All of these properties are dependent on balloon composition. Modern balloons are composed of polyethylene, polyolefin copolymer, nylon, or polyethylene terephthalate.[3] Each material confers different characteristics to the balloon, the most important of which is compliance. Noncompliant balloons reach their nominal diameter early in the inflation period and thereafter tolerate greater pressures without changing diameter. The net effect is to transmit the increased pressure force more equally and radially throughout the lesion. Conversely, compliant balloons will continue to stretch with increasing balloon pressure, often beyond its nominal diameter, leading to uneven pressure transmission in mixed soft/hard lesions with associated overstretched/understretched areas of lesion, respectively. Figures 4.17 and 4.18 further illustrate the property of compliance.

Table 4.12 summarizes the two main catheter platform systems that are available and their associated clinical advantages and disadvantages. Figure 4.19 illustrates the particular design specifications.

Balloon Catheter Selection

Tables 4.13 and 4.14 describe different types of compliant and noncompliant balloons and their respective clinical indications.

After selecting the appropriate balloon type and platform[9], the appropriate balloon size is picked in relation to the vessel size at a ratio of 0.75–1.1:1.0.

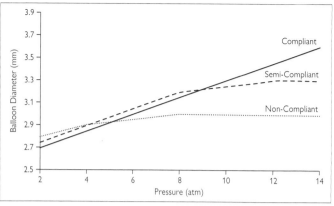

Figure 4.17 Balloon compliance. Reprinted from Holmes DR, Mathew V. *Atlas of interventional cardiology*, 2nd ed. Philadelphia: Current Medicine, Inc., 2003, with permission of the publisher (Current Medicine Group LLC).

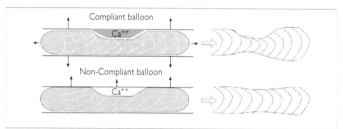

Figure 4.18 Compliance and outcomes on calcified lesions. Reproduced from Werns SW, Topol EJ. Review of Hardware of PTCA. *Journal of Interventional Cardiology* 1988;1:209-19. With permission from publisher (Wiley-Blackwell).

Table 4.12 Comparison of over-the-wire versus rapid-exchange balloon dilatation catheters

	Design	Advantages	Disadvantages
Over-the-wire (OTW)	Movable guidewire runs through a central lumen which runs the entire length of catheter	• Useful for lesions requiring multiple balloon exchanges (e.g., chronic total occlusions) • Allows better "push" of balloon due to wire support throughout entire length of catheter	• Two operators needed • Requires exchange length wires • Requires balloon catheter shaft to be larger
Rapid-exchange (RX)	Movable guidewire runs through a central lumen which runs from tip of catheter and then exits just distal to the balloon.	• Single operator • Simpler to use • Allows for smaller sized catheter shafts	• Cannot be used easily for lesions requiring wire exchanges via balloon catheter

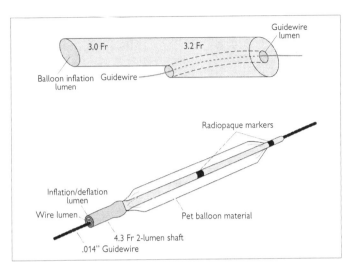

Figure 4.19 Comparison of RX balloon catheter (*top*) versus over-the-wire system (*bottom*).

Table 4.13 Commonly used balloon catheters

Noncompliant	Compliant/Semicompliant
Quantum Maverick	Maverick
Voyager noncompliant	Voyager
Merlin	Apex

Table 4.14 Indications for compliant/semicompliant versus noncompliant balloons

	Advantages	Disadvantages
Noncompliant	• Useful for calcified lesions by directing radial force against lesion • Useful for postdilation of stents to ensure full stent strut apposition • Useful for long lesions	• Harder to deliver due to larger profile and stiffer construction • If lesion size underestimated, upsizing requires placing new balloon
Semicompliant/ Compliant	• Decreased profile improves deliverability • Suitable for noncalcified or ACS lesions • Useful for situations where target lesion size uncertain; can inflate to desired size	• In calcified lesions, balloon will overstretch soft portions of artery predisposing to dissection

Cutting Balloons

The cutting balloon (Boston Scientific, Natick, MA) is a noncompliant balloon that is mounted with three or four microtomes positioned in a longitudinal manner[3] (Fig. 4.20). Clinical indications and contraindications for the use of cutting balloons are summarized in Table 4.15.

If a cutting balloon is used, a 7 or 8 Fr guide catheter should be employed, and a negative prep should be used to keep the blades withdrawn at all times until ready for inflation. The inflation and deflation rates should be slow, as this decreases chances of coronary perforation.

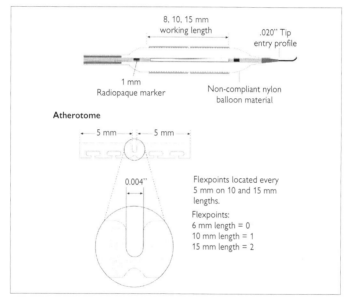

Figure 4.20 Cutting balloon. From http://www.bostonscientific.com/Device. bsci?page=HCP_Overview&navRelId=1000.1003&method=DevDetailHCP&id=10004791 &pageDisclaimer=Disclaimer.ProductPage
Reproduced with permission from Boston Scientific, 2009.

Table 4.15 Cutting balloon use

Indications	Contraindications
Moderately calcified lesions	Heavily calcified lesion/vessel → rotational atherectomy should be used instead
Ostial lesions	Severely angulated lesion → risk of perforation too high
In-stent restenosis → minimizes slippage of balloon during angioplasty (watermelon seed effect)	Very tortuous vessel → risk of perforation too high
Bifurcations lesions → minimizes plaque shift during balloon inflation/stent placement	Patient cannot tolerate slow inflation/ deflation rates

Practical Pearls

- Selecting the appropriate guiding catheter, guidewire, and balloon catheter for each case is key to technical success.

- The best approach to guidewire choice is to select a "workhorse" wire for several case scenarios and become thoroughly familiar with the selected wire's behavior.

- Noncompliant balloons are useful for calcified lesions and for postdilation of stents to ensure full stent strut apposition.

- A cutting balloon is useful for moderately calcified lesions, but is not recommended for severely calcified lesions.

References

1. Nguyen TN, Colombo A, Hu D, Grines CL, Saito S. *Practical handbook of advanced interventional cardiology*, 3rd. New York: Wiley-Blackwell, 2007.

2. Ikari Y, Nagaoka M, Kim JY, Morino Y, Tanabe T. The physics of guiding catheters for the left coronary artery in transfemoral and transradial interventions. *J Invasive Cardiol.* 2005;17:636-641.

3. Holmes DR, Mathew V. *Atlas of interventional cardiology*, 2nd ed. Philadelphia: Current Medicine, Inc., 2003.

4. Ellis SG, Holmes DR. *Strategic approaches in coronary intervention*, 3rd ed. Philadelphia: Lippincott Williams & Wilkins, 2006.

5. Cordis Corporation. *Cordis VistaBrite Tip: Shapes for variable take-offs*. Johnson & Johnson, 2007.

6. Douglas JS. Selection and use of basic equipment, guiding catheters, wires, and balloons. In: Kern MJ, Berger PB, Block PC, Klein L, Laskey W, eds. *SCAI interventional cardiology board review book*. Philadelphia: Lippincott Williams & Wilkins, 2006.

7. Avedissian MG, Killeavy ES, Garcia JM, Dear WE. Percutaneous transluminal coronary angioplasty: a review of current balloon dilatation systems. *Cathet Cardiovasc Diagn.* 1989;18:263-275.

8. Werns SW, Topol EJ. Review of hardware of PTCA. *J Intervent Cardiol.* 1988;1: 209-219.

9. Balloon and wires: "Still the staples of PCI." Henry Ford Vascular Institute, n.d. Accessed November 20, 2009 at http://www.cardiosource.com/img/FB_Balloons_and_Wires.ppt

Chapter 5

Coronary Artery Stenting

Henry Roukoz

The benefit derived from balloon angioplasty in coronary artery disease is limited by early vessel closure and late neointimal hyperplasia. The advent of stents has dropped acute vessel closure to less than 1%, subacute thrombosis to about 1%, and subsequent need for revascularization to about 20% with bare metal stents (BMSs) and 10% with drug-eluting stents (DESs).[1] Stenting is now the most common modality of revascularization in patients with coronary artery disease and is performed in the vast majority of percutaneous coronary interventions (PCIs).

This chapter reviews stent design and properties; commercially available stents; the stenting procedure with focus on stent choice, advancement, and deployment; direct stenting; and finally, adjuvant pharmacotherapy.

Stent Design

Clinically Relevant Stent Properties

Ideally, stent design should optimize the following characteristics:[2]

- *Good trackability and longitudinal flexibility*: These two properties enable the stent to cross angulated or tortuous segments and reach the target lesion without stent dislodgement, intimal injury, or vasospasm.
- *High radial strength and low intrinsic recoil*: Once deployed, the stent must resist the acute elastic recoil of the media and surrounding plaque. This will also help to seal the entry point of a dissection.
- *Good conformability*: This property gives the stent the ability to conform to a curved or tortuous segment after deployment, molding its shape while keeping a good apposition to the vessel wall, and without forcing its original straight shape on the segment.
- *Low metallic surface area*: This minimizes contact of metal with both the intima and the blood, theoretically decreasing early and late stent thrombosis.
- *Biocompatibility*: This minimizes the inflammation or allergic reaction to the stent, which have been implicated in stent restenosis and thrombosis.

- *Radiographic visibility*: Adequate radiopacity will help visualize the stent during deployment, without obscuring luminal details.

Composition

Other than the documented effect of gold on actually increasing restenosis compared with stainless steel,[3,4] there are only theoretical advantages of one type of metal over the other. Moreover, surface texture and finishing may affect stent thrombosis or restenosis.[5]

- *316L stainless steel*: The most common metal used for balloon-expandable stents. This alloy contains mainly iron and 16% chromium, making it biologically inert, but it also contains 10%–14% nickel (a potential source of allergic reactions) and 2%–3% molybdenum.

- *Cobalt/platinum and cobalt/chromium alloys*: These alloys allow thin stent struts without sacrificing strength. They are more radiopaque, and may elicit less host response, than stainless steel.

- *Biodegradable polymer-based and magnesium-based stents*: Theoretically, these may reduce late stent thrombosis, and they can facilitate subsequent revascularization at the price of reduced radial strength and decreased radiopacity.

Configuration

Stents can be classified into three general configurations:

- *Wire coil*: Constructed by shaping a stainless steel nanofilament into reversing loops to form an expandable interdigitating coil. This design has low radial strength and a tendency for plaque to prolapse between adjacent loops, due to large gaps after deployment, thus causing more acute vessel closure and late restenosis. Subsequently, this design fell out of favor.

- *Tubular and multicellular design*: The tubular design consists of a metal tube with laser-cut rectangular or curved slots that will open into a diamond or circular shape when expanded, giving it good radial strength and wall coverage at the price of lower crossing flexibility and varying side branch accessibility. The shorter, thinner, and more interrupted the struts are, the more flexible the stent. The more circumferentially the struts move after expansion, the more radial strength. The multicellular design consists of varying cell shapes and sizes along the stent (*open-cell* design) or a repeated pattern of uniform cells (*closed-cell* design), increasing flexibility, trackability, and side branch access without sacrificing radial strength. Closed-cell designs tend to have better wall coverage and less flexibility than open-cell designs.

- *Modular or hybrid design*: To further increase flexibility while keeping the advantages of the tubular design, the hybrid design joins multiple modules of varying lengths and strut profiles. This confers increased wall coverage and crossing profile, and decreases design trade-offs.

Covered stents are metallic stents covered with a microporous polytetrafluoroethylene (PTFE) membrane. They are mainly used to treat coronary perforations, cover aneurysms, and close fistulas. They have an increased risk of restenosis and thrombosis.

Components of a Drug-eluting Stent

Drug-eluting stents have three components: a *stent platform*, a *bioactive agent* to reduce neointimal hyperplasia, and a *drug carrier* to control the dosing and release of the bioactive agent. Drug-eluting stents should ideally achieve homogeneous and controlled drug delivery to avoid subtherapeutic doses in one spot and toxic doses in others. Closed-cell designs tend to have more uniform coverage and subsequently more homogenous drug delivery. The most frequently used stents are presented in Tables 5.1 and 5.2.

Stenting Procedure

Choosing Stent Length and Diameter

- *Choosing the optimal length*: The stent should be able to cover the whole lesion, starting approximately 2 mm before and 2 mm after the lesion, to minimize edge dissection and ensure a smooth transition form proximal normal segment to distal normal segment. Excessively long stents covering angiographically normal segments should be avoided, given the increased risk of thrombosis and restenosis.[6,7] Use one long stent for a long lesion if possible. If more than one is necessary, the stents should overlap by about 2 mm to ensure adequate coverage. In a diffusely diseased vessel, it is preferable to stent distal to proximal to ensure complete lesion coverage (i.e., complete stent delivery).

- *Choosing the optimal diameter*: The diameter of the stent should optimally correspond to the reference vessel diameter in a nondiseased segment. Intravascular ultrasound (IVUS) is useful for more precisely determining the reference vessel diameter. Both under- and oversizing the stent can result in adverse outcomes.

Table 5.1 Most commonly used bare metal stents

Characteristics	Liberté	Multi-Link Vision Multi-Link Mini Vision	Driver Micro-Driver
Manufacturer	Boston Scientific	Abbott	Medtronic
Composition	316L Stainless Steel	L605 Cobalt-Chromium	MP35N Cobalt-Nickel
Strut size	.0038"	.0032"	.0036"
Diameters available	2.75, 3.0, 3.5, 4.0, 4.5, 5.0	Multi-Link Vision: 2.75, 3.0, 3.5, 4.0 Multi-Link Mini Vision: 2.0, 2.25, 2.5	Driver: 3.0, 3.5, 4.0 Micro-Driver: 2.25, 2.5, 2.75
Lengths available	8, 12, 16, 20, 24, 28, 32	8, 12, 15, 18, 23, 28	Driver: 9, 12, 15, 18, 24, 30 Micro-Driver: 8, 12, 14, 18, 24

Table 5.2 The most commonly used drug–eluting stents

Characteristics	Cypher	Taxus Express	Taxus Liberté	Xience V Promus	Endeavor
BMS[1] platform	Bx Velocity	Express	Liberté	Multi-Link Vision Multi-Link Mini Vision	Driver Micro-Driver
Manufacturer	Cordis Corporation Johnson & Johnson	Boston Scientific		Boston Scientific Abbott	
Composition	316L Stainless Steel	316L Stainless Steel	316L Stainless Steel	L605 Cobalt-Chromium	MP35N Cobalt-Nickel
Strut size	.0055"	.0052"	.0038"	.0032"	.0036"
Bioactive agent	Sirolimus	Paclitaxel	Paclitaxel	Everolimus	Zatrolimus
Polymer design	Dual layer over primer	Single layer	Single layer over primer	Single layer over primer	Single layer over primer with overspray
Carrier/polymer with layer composition	**Primer:** Parylene C **Layer 1:** Sirolimus + PEVA[2] and PBMA[3] **Layer 2:** PBMA[3]	**Layer 1:** Translute (Paclitaxel + SIBS[4])		**Primer:** PBMA[3] **Layer 1:** Everolimus + Fluorinated co-polymer	**Primer:** PC[5] **Layer 1:** Zatrolimus + PC[5] **Overspray:** PC[5]
Drug release	Fast (~80% at 30 days)	Slow (~8% at 30 days)		Fast (~70% at 30 days)	Fast (~100% at 30 days)
Diameters available (millimeters)	2.5, 2.75, 3.0, 3.5	Taxus Express: 2.5, 2.75, 3.0, 3.5 Taxus Express Atom: 2.25	Taxus Liberté: 2.5, 2.75, 3.0, 3.5, 4.0 Taxus Liberté Atom: 2.25	2.5, 2.75, 3.0, 3.5, 4.0	2.5, 3.0, 3.5
Lengths available (millimeters)	8, 13, 18, 23, 28, 33	Taxus Express: 8, 12, 16, 20, 24, 28, 32 Taxus Express Atom: 8, 12, 16, 20, 24	8, 12, 16, 20, 24, 28, 32	8, 12, 15, 18, 23, 28	8, 9, 12, 14, 15, 18, 24, 30

1. Bare metal stent; 2. polyethylene–co–vinyl acetate; 3. poly N-butyl methacrylate; 4. poly(styrene-b-isobutylene-b-styrene); 5. phosphorylcholine.

Stent Advancement

Stent advancement is affected by the stability and backup of the guiding cathe-ter, the stiffness of the wire, and the tortuosity of the vessel. In case of difficulty with advancing a stent, the following methods could be attempted:

- *Guide*: Manipulate the guide into a more stable position:
  - Deep-seat the guide (only with experienced operators due to risk of dissection)
  - Upsize the guiding catheter (e.g., 7 or 8 Fr) or change the guide (e.g., Amplatz guiding catheter) for extra backup.
- *Wire*: Pull the wire back minimally while advancing the stent to facilitate stent advancement:
  - Add an extra support wire (e.g., Iron Man or Grand Slam) to straighten the artery.
- *Balloon*: Inflate another balloon distal to the target lesion, thus jailing the guidewire; pull the wire slightly to put tension on it; and advance the stent. However, this is not optimal due to risk of restenosis from the angioplastied segment.
- *Stent*: Choose a more flexible stent. Current-generation DES are more deliv-erable than first-generation DES; however, a BMS is even more deliverable.
  - Use two shorter stents instead of one long one to cover the lesion.

Stent Deployment

- *Positioning*: The stent should optimally cover the entire lesion. In tortuous ves-sels, the positioning of the proximal or distal edge of the stent at an angulated segment should be avoided, since this might make recrossing or postdilation difficult and might promote restenosis. In these cases, deploying the stent while the patient is taking a deep breath will make the heart more vertical and the artery curvature straighter and more elongated. It is especially important to ask the patient to stop breathing during deployment from the radial approach, since breathing movements can induce greater guide movements than the femoral approach.
- *Optimal pressure*: The nominal pressure expands the stent to its prespecified (or nominal) diameter ± 10% (Table 5.3). The rated burst pressure (RBP) is the maximum pressure that the stent balloon can safely withstand before rupturing. The goal is to use a high enough pressure to achieve full apposi-tion of the stent to the vessel wall without causing dissection at the edge of the stent or strut fracture. The optimal pressure should be dictated by vessel anatomy. High pressures (16–18 atm) may be needed with a slightly undersized stent or calcified lesion to ensure complete stent expansion and apposition to the vessel wall. In contrast, lower pressures (11–14 atm) may suffice in other circumstances.
- *Optimal inflation time*: This parameter is not well evaluated; however, most inflation times range from 15 to 60 seconds.[8,9]

Table 5.3 Balloon pressure for stent deployment

Inflation Pressure (atm)	Stent Size (mm)	
6	2.17	
7	2.25	
8	2.32	
9	2.38	
10	2.44	
11	**2.49**	**Nominal** Balloon pressure to get to designed diameter
12	2.53	
13	2.56	
14	2.59	
15	2.62	
16	**2.64**	**RBP** Rated Burst Pressure
17	2.67	**Risk of strut fracture**
18	2.69	
19	2.73	
20	2.74	

This an example of a typical compliance table that comes with each stent brand and size. Pressures beyond the rated burst pressure (RBP) are not recommended due to risk of strut fracture.

- *Postdilation*: In general, postdilation is a good strategy to ensure complete stent expansion and apposition to the vessel wall, especially when used with IVUS guidance. If the vessel is tapering, the proximal segment of the stent might not be fully apposed to the vessel wall and can be expanded further using a larger noncompliant balloon with higher pressure, covering only the proximal to mid segments of the stent. In diffusely diseased vessels, a stent can be deployed with moderate pressures to avoid edge dissection then postdilated with a higher pressure and a shorter noncompliant balloon kept within the margins of the stent.

- *Use of IVUS and functional flow reserver (FFR)*: Intravenous ultrasound measurements prior to (to choose adequate stent size) and after (to ensure expansion and apposition) stent implantation have improved outcomes. Physiologic assessment with functional flow reserve (FFR) is used to assess the need for intervention (FFR <0.75–0.80) and determine the adequacy of stent implantation (FFR<0.95 correlates with stent underdeployment by IVUS).[10,11]

- *Optimal angiographic result*: The aim is to have a residual stenosis of less than 10%, no edge dissection, a TIMI 3 flow, side branch patency with a diameter greater than 2 mm, and the absence of electrocardiographic changes, symptoms, or hemodynamic instability.

Direct Stenting Versus Predilation Balloon Angioplasty

Direct stenting reduces procedure time and cost, fluoroscopy time, and contrast use, and it has equivalent early and late outcomes compared to predilation.[12,13] However, forceful manipulation should be avoided when crossing a tight or calcified lesion because of the risk of damaging or stripping the stent off its balloon, thus causing stent embolization or vessel thrombosis due to endothelial or plaque injury. In these cases, predilation should be attempted before readvancing the stent. Predilation is also favored in total occlusion, bifurcation lesions, long lesions, proximal tortuosity, and distal vessel lesions. A down-side of predilation is the potential for geographic miss if an angioplastied segment is not stented.

Drug-eluting Stent Versus Bare Metal Stent

Drug-eluting stents significantly decrease revascularization rates compared to BMSs, although first-generation DESs have been shown to increase late stent thrombosis.[1,14] It is uncertain if second-generation DESs carry the same increased risk for late thrombosis compared with BMSs. Bare metal stents are still favored when patients have an anticipated surgery, low compliance to medication, or history of bleeding because they require shorter double antiplatelet therapy.[15]

Adjuvant Pharmacotherapy[16]

Aspirin

- All patients should have at least 325 mg of aspirin at least 2 hours before PCI (Class I).

Clopidogrel

- A loading dose of 300–600 mg of clopidogrel should be given prior to PCI (Class I).
- If clopidogrel is given at the time of PCI and not before PCI, a glycoprotein IIb/IIIa inhibitor can be considered (Class IIa).

Glycoprotein IIb/IIIa Inhibitors

- Should be administered in patients with unstable angina/non-ST segment elevation myocardial infarction (UA/NSTEMI) *without* clopidogrel administration (abciximab, eptifibatide, or tirofiban) (Class I).
- Reasonable in patients with UA/NSTEMI *with* clopidogrel administration (abciximab, eptifibatide, or tirofiban) (Class IIa).
- Reasonable in patients with STEMI undergoing PCI (abciximab) (Class IIa).
- Reasonable in patients undergoing elective PCI (abciximab, eptifibatide, or tirofiban). This is often in a "bail-out" situation (Class IIa).

Heparin/Antithrombotic Therapy

- An antithrombin agent (for example, unfractionated heparin or bivalirudin) should be administered to patients undergoing PCI (Class I).

- For patients with heparin-induced thrombocytopenia, it is recommended that bivalirudin or argatroban be used to replace heparin (Class I).

- Low-molecular-weight heparin can be considered an alternative to unfractionated heparin in patients with UA/NSTEMI undergoing PCI (Class IIa).

- In patients *without* a glycoprotein IIb/IIIa inhibitor, give heparin 70–100 IU/kg bolus (maximum 4,000 IU) to achieve activated coagulation time (ACT) of 250–300 sec with the HemoTec device and 300–350 sec with the Hemochron device.

- In patients *with* glycoprotein IIb/IIIa inhibitor, give heparin bolus of 50–60 IU/kg and target an ACT of 200–250 sec with either the HemoTec or Hemochron device.

Emerging Therapies

- *New coatings*: Fully biodegradable polymers like polylactic acid (PLA) and polylactic-co-glycolic acid (PLGA) are being investigated. Other designs avoid polymers completely and use a cover of titanium-nitric oxide alloy.

- *New drugs*: These include tacrolimus, pimecrolimus, biolimus, murine monoclonal anti-CD34 antibodies, the anti–vascular endothelial growth factor (VEGF) bevacizumab, and genistein, a natural isoflavonoid phytoestrogen.

- *Fully bioabsorbable stents*: These aim to decrease late stent thrombosis and the need for prolonged antiplatelet therapy, restore vasoreactivity, and make subsequent percutaneous or surgical revascularization easier. They include an everolimus-eluting PLA stent (BVS; Abbott Laboratories, IL),[17] a tyrosine-derived polycarbonate REVA stent (REVA medical, San Diego, CA), and a biolimus-A9-eluting biodegradable PLA stent (BioMatrix Flex, Biosensors Inc., Newport Beach, CA).[18]

Practical Pearls

- The ideal stent characteristics include longitudinal flexibility and high radial strength. The new hybrid stent designs tend to minimize trade-offs.

- Anticoagulate with heparin for a goal ACT of 250–300 sec. Load with aspirin (325 mg) and clopidogrel (300–600 mg) before the procedure. Glycoprotein IIb/IIIa inhibitors can be considered in acute coronary syndromes and for "bail-out" in elective PCI.

- Advance the stent gently to avoid vasospasm and intimal injury. The entire lesion should be covered. Use moderate to high balloon pressure and post-dilation if needed to ensure complete apposition.

- Predilation is favored in long or tight calcified lesions, total occlusion, bifurcation lesions, proximal tortuosity, and distal vessel lesions.

- Routinely establish arterial or venous access with the micropuncture needle to minimize bleeding complications.

- Before performing PCI, always check an ACT to ensure that the antithrombin agent is producing an effect. This safeguards against the occasionally infiltrated peripheral intravenous line.
- Rotational atherectomy should be performed if there is inability to reduce a lesion with balloon dilatation. Once a stent is deployed in a nonreducible stenosis, it may be impossible to reduce the lesion even with high-pressure balloon inflation.
- An over-the-wire balloon can be removed from a short wire by the hydraulic technique. In this technique, the balloon shaft is railed back (keeping the wire fixed in place) until the wire is within the balloon shaft. Then, a high-pressure syringe filled with saline is attached to the hub of the balloon shaft and injected while gently pulling back. This will leave the wire in place, while removing the balloon from the body.
- An additional technique to facilitate stent delivery is the use of the Wiggle Wire. This can be especially helpful when trying to navigate around a previously placed stent.
- After stent deployment, final angiographic images should include two orthogonal views with the guidewire removed. This helps to detect edge dissections.

References

1. Roukoz H, Bavry AA, Sarkees ML, et al. Comprehensive meta-analysis on drug-eluting stents versus bare-metal stents during extended follow-up. *Am J Med.* 2009;122:581.e1-581.e10.

2. Rieu R, Barragan P, Garitey V, et al. Assessment of the trackability, flexibility, and conformability of coronary stents: a comparative analysis. *Catheter Cardiovasc Interv.* 2003;59:496-503.

3. Reifart N, Morice MC, Silber S, et al. The NUGGET study: NIR ultra gold-gilded equivalency trial. *Catheter Cardiovasc Interv.* 2004;62:18-25.

4. Kastrati A, Schomig A, Dirschinger J, et al. Increased risk of restenosis after placement of gold-coated stents: results of a randomized trial comparing gold-coated with uncoated steel stents in patients with coronary artery disease. *Circulation.* 2000;101:2478-2483.

5. Hehrlein C, Zimmermann M, Metz J, Ensinger W, Kubler W. Influence of surface texture and charge on the biocompatibility of endovascular stents. *Coronary Artery Dis.* 1995;6:581-586.

6. Moreno R, Fernandez C, Hernandez R, et al. Drug-eluting stent thrombosis: results from a pooled analysis including 10 randomized studies. *J Am Coll Cardiol.* 2005;45:954-959.

7. Machecourt J, Danchin N, Lablanche JM, et al. Risk factors for stent thrombosis after implantation of sirolimus-eluting stents in diabetic and nondiabetic patients: the EVASTENT Matched-Cohort Registry. *J Am Coll Cardiol.* 2007;50:501-508.

8. Trindade IS, Sarmento-Leite R, Santos de Freitas M, Gottschall CA. Determination of the minimum inflation time necessary for total stent expansion and apposition: an in vitro study. *J Invasive Cardiol.* 2008;20:396-398.

9. Kawasaki T, Koga H, Serikawa T, et al. Impact of a prolonged delivery inflation time for optimal drug-eluting stent expansion. *Catheter Cardiovasc Interv.* 2009;73:205-211.

10. Pijls NH, van Schaardenburgh P, Manoharan G, et al. Percutaneous coronary intervention of functionally nonsignificant stenosis: 5-year follow-up of the DEFER Study. *J Am Coll Cardiol.* 2007;49:2105-2111.

11. Tonino PA, De Bruyne B, Pijls NH, et al. Fractional flow reserve versus angiography for guiding percutaneous coronary intervention. *N Engl J Med.* 2009;360:213-224.

12. Ormiston JA, Mahmud E, Turco MA, et al. Direct stenting with the TAXUS Liberte drug-eluting stent: results from the Taxus Atlas Direct Stent Study. *JACC Cardiovasc Intervent.* 2008;1:150-160.

13. Schluter M, Schofer J, Gershlick AH, et al. Direct stenting of native de novo coronary artery lesions with the sirolimus-eluting stent: a post hoc subanalysis of the pooled E- and C-SIRIUS trials. *J Am Coll Cardiol.* 2005;45:10-13.

14. Bavry AA, Kumbhani DJ, Helton TJ, Borek PP, Mood GR, Bhatt DL. Late thrombosis of drug-eluting stents: a meta-analysis of randomized clinical trials. *Am J Med.* 2006;119:1056-1061.

15. Bavry AA, Bhatt DL. Appropriate use of drug-eluting stents: balancing the reduction in restenosis with the concern of late thrombosis. *Lancet.* 2008;371:2134-2143.

16. King SB, 3rd, Smith SC, Jr., Hirshfeld JW, Jr., et al. 2007 focused update of the ACC/AHA/SCAI 2005 guideline update for percutaneous coronary intervention: a report of the American College of Cardiology/American Heart Association Task Force on Practice guidelines. *J Am Coll Cardiol.* 2008;51:172-209.

17. Serruys PW, Ormiston JA, Onuma Y, et al. A bioabsorbable everolimus-eluting coronary stent system (ABSORB): 2-year outcomes and results from multiple imaging methods. *Lancet.* 2009;373:897-910.

18. Windecker S, Serruys PW, Wandel S, et al. Biolimus-eluting stent with biodegradable polymer versus sirolimus-eluting stent with durable polymer for coronary revascularisation (LEADERS): a randomised non-inferiority trial. *Lancet.* 2008;372:1163-1173.

Chapter 6

Coronary Flow Reserve, Fractional Flow Reserve, Intravascular Ultrasound, and Optical Coherence Tomography

Adnan K. Chhatriwalla

Coronary angiography and percutaneous coronary intervention (PCI) have revolutionized cardiovascular medicine. Nevertheless, the limitations of coronary angiography are well recognized. Coronary angiography provides information only on the patency of the arterial lumen, and it may be limited by spatial resolution as well as by difficulties in visualization due to vessel tortuosity, overlapping branches, vessel calcification, and eccentric plaque. Large intra- and interobserver variability exists in the angiographic assessment of stenosis severity. Furthermore, clinical symptoms are dependent on coronary blood flow, which is not directly measured by coronary angiography. In this chapter, we review techniques developed to complement the information obtained by coronary angiography, in order to improve visualization and better assess lesion severity.

Coronary and Fractional Flow Reserve

Coronary flow reserve (CFR) and fractional flow reserve (FFR) are invasive indices of the physiologic significance of a coronary stenosis. The development of ultra-thin Doppler and pressure angioplasty guidewires in the early 1990s allowed for the measurement of velocity and pressure in the coronary arteries and the physiologic assessment of coronary stenoses in humans. Doppler-derived flow index was first described as the ratio of blood velocity in a vessel distal to an occluded balloon, to blood velocity in the same vessel during patency. Subsequently, the use of coronary pressure to assess the contribution of epicardial flow to a given coronary bed was described. Both calculations are based on the premise that blood flow is proportional to velocity and pressure when vessel surface area is constant and both Doppler-derived and pressure-derived flow indices have been clinically validated.

Coronary flow reserve calculation is performed using a wire with a piezo-electric ultrasound crystal at its tip that measures blood flow velocity by tim-ing the return of ultrasound waves reflected off of red blood cells. Coronary flow reserve is calculated as the ratio of hyperemic to basal coronary flow. A normal CFR is 3.0–5.0, and a CFR of less than 2.0 is indicative of a flow-limiting epicardial coronary artery stenosis or microvascular disease, and it corresponds to myocardial ischemia as diagnosed by noninvasive functional studies.[1] Furthermore, improvement in CFR following angioplasty has been shown to predict long-term clinical success. In the DEBATE study, patients achieving a CFR of greater than 2.5 and residual diameter stenosis of greater than 35% after balloon angioplasty had lower rates of restenosis (16% vs. 41%), need for intervention (16% vs. 34%), and recurrence of symptoms at 6 months (23% vs. 47%).[2]

Fractional flow reserve is defined as the maximal achievable flow in a myo-cardial bed in the presence of a stenosis divided by the maximal flow through the same bed in the theoretic absence of the stenosis. Fractional flow reserve is simply measured as the mean intracoronary pressure distal to a lesion divided by the mean aortic pressure during maximal hyperemia. A normal FFR is 1.0, and an FFR value of less than 0.75 has been shown to be highly predictive of ischemia on noninvasive testing in patients with coronary artery disease.[3] Unlike CFR, which takes into account the epicardial and microvascular circulation, FFR reflects the physiological significance of an epicardial coronary artery stenosis while minimizing the contribution of the microvascular circulation. Nonetheless, it has been theorized that the presence of microvascular coronary artery dis-ease, as in diabetes, left ventricular hypertrophy, or acute myocardial infarction (MI), may limit maximal microvascular vasodilatation and thus render FFR cal-culation less precise.[4] However, whether these theoretic concerns significantly limit the clinical value of FFR is not clear.[5]

The DEFER study demonstrated that patients with intermediate angio-graphic coronary stenosis and an FFR of more than 0.75 had no benefit from PCI in terms of death, MI, need for bypass surgery, or need for repeat coronary intervention at 5 years.[6] More recently, the FAME study demonstrated that FFR-guided PCI, using a threshold of 0.80, reduced the risk of death or MI by 35%, and death, MI, or repeat revascularization by 30% when compared to angiography-guided PCI.[7] Fractional flow reserve can also be used to evaluate the success of a PCI procedure. Following PCI, the translesional gradient should decrease, and a post-PCI FFR value of greater than 0.90 is considered optimal.

Coronary Flow Reserve Procedure

Following anticoagulant administration, a 0.014-inch Doppler wire is advanced through the guide catheter approximately 2 cm distal to the lesion identified by angiography. The system is connected to a real-time spectrum analyzer, which measures coronary blood flow velocity. Flow velocity is measured con-tinuously at baseline and at maximal hyperemia, following the administration of intracoronary adenosine (24–72 μg) or papaverine (10–12 mg). The CFR is calculated as the ratio of peak hyperemic to basal coronary blood flow velocity.

Fractional Flow Reserve Procedure

The 0.014-inch pressure-monitoring wire is placed in saline flush, and the pressure is zeroed outside the body. Following anticoagulant administration, the wire is advanced from the guide catheter such that the transducer on the pressure wire (approximately 3 cm proximal to the tip and at the radiopaque junction) is at the tip of the guiding catheter and equalized to aortic pressure, as measured through the guiding catheter. The transducer is then advanced distal to the lesion identified by angiography so that the pressure transducer is beyond the lesion. Hyperemia is then induced by administration of intravenous (140 μg/kg/min) or intracoronary adenosine (24–72 μg), or intracoronary papaverine (10–12 mg). The intravenous route of vasodilator administration is preferred, as it allows for more stable and predictable microvascular dilatation. Measurements of distal intracoronary pressure (P_d) and aortic pressure (P_{Ao}) are then continuously recorded, and FFR is calculated as the ratio of P_d to P_{Ao} during maximal hyperemia (Fig. 6.1). Post procedure, the pressure wire and guiding catheter pressures should be rechecked with the wire at the tip of the catheter (the pressures should be equal) to assure absence of signal drift.

Intravascular Ultrasound

Intravascular ultrasound (IVUS) utilizes a catheter with an ultrasound probe at its tip to provide a two-dimensional cross-sectional image of the coronary artery. Whereas coronary angiography only provides information regarding the patency of the arterial lumen, IVUS allows visualization of the arterial lumen, as well as the arterial wall, in three layers: intima, media, and adventitia (Fig. 6.2).

Lumen cross-sectional area (CSA) may be measured directly from IVUS still frames, and CSA measurements of less than 3.0 mm^2 in the major epicardial vessels or less than 6.0–7.5 mm^2 in the left main coronary artery have been correlated with physiologically significant stenoses as measured by FFR.[8,9] IVUS may be used to calculate atheroma volume, which has been used as a surrogate endpoint for the study of antiatherosclerotic therapies, by subtracting the luminal CSA from the area bounded by the external elastic membrane (Fig. 6.2). Furthermore, IVUS has been used in the visualization of plaque components (including fibrous cap, lipid core, and calcium), and may it assist in the identification of plaques vulnerable to rupture.[10]

IVUS may be used to optimize the results of PCI by accurately measuring vessel diameter and lesion length to assist in proper balloon and stent sizing. Furthermore, IVUS can aid in the visualization of side branches and previously deployed stents, and it can identify lesion characteristics that may guide the use of specialized interventional techniques, such as the use of rotational atherectomy in heavily calcified lesions or directional atherectomy in bifurcation lesions or lesions with a large plaque burden. Finally, IVUS may identify

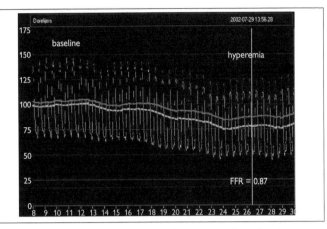

Figure 6.1 A screen shot demonstrating simultaneous recordings of aortic pressure and post-stenotic arterial pressure used to calculate fractional flow reserve (FFR). In this case, the FFR was 0.87 at maximal hyperemia, indicating a non–flow limiting stenosis.

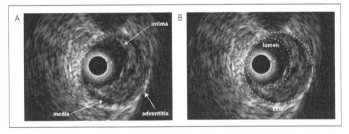

Figure 6.2 An intravascular ultrasound (IVUS) still frame depicting atherosclerosis. In A, the three layers of the arterial wall are labeled. In B, the arterial lumen is the area located within the inner dotted line, whereas the external elastic membrane (EEM) is the circumference delineated by outer dotted line. The area between the arterial lumen and the EEM represents atherosclerotic plaque.

suboptimal PCI results, such as residual dissection, stent underexpansion, or stent malapposition, which require further attention. The results of the MUSIC study demonstrated an impressive 8.3% rate of angiographic restenosis at 6 months in patients treated with IVUS-guided stenting.[11] Similarly, the CRUISE study suggested a 44% decrease in target vessel revascularization at 9 months in patients treated with IVUS-guided stenting (8.5% vs. 15.3%).[12] However, other studies of IVUS-guided stenting strategies have demonstrated mixed results.

Intravascular Ultrasound Procedure

Two types of IVUS catheters are available: *mechanical catheters*, which rotate to visualize the entire vessel, and *phased-array catheters*, which use multiple transducers positioned around the circumference of the catheter to visualize the entire vessel. Both types of catheters should be flushed prior to use. Mechanical catheters rotate, advance, and retract inside a telescoping shaft, which must be flushed with heparinized saline prior to use. Phased-array catheters require flushing of the wire lumen. Following anticoagulant administration, the IVUS catheter is advanced into the coronary artery over a wire in monorail fashion. Intracoronary nitroglycerin (50–200 μg) should be administered to promote vasodilatation prior to image acquisition and to prevent arterial spasm. Cross-sectional images of the coronary artery may be obtained at a fixed rate during slow manual or mechanical pullback of the IVUS catheter through the coronary segment of interest. Image acquisition can be performed as the catheter is advanced (proximal to distal in the coronary artery) or as the catheter is pulled back (distal to proximal).

Optical Coherence Tomography

Optical coherence tomography (OCT) utilizes fiberoptic technology to visualize the coronary artery. Optical coherence tomography generates images from reflected electromagnetic waves emitted from a light source, rather than from ultrasound waves, as in IVUS. Light in the near-infrared range, with a wavelength of approximately 1,300 nm is used. As a result, tremendous spatial resolution is possible with OCT, on the order of 4–16 μm, compared to 100–150 μm with IVUS.[13] However, this improved spatial resolution comes at the expense of a limited tissue penetration depth of only 2–3 mm. Therefore, OCT imaging is typically limited beyond the internal elastic lamina, and it cannot be used to fully evaluate the extent of atherosclerosis in the arterial wall or to quantify plaque volume. Nonetheless, image acquisition times are very rapid (4–15 frames/sec), thus allowing for high-resolution imaging of the near field without significant motion artifact.

As with IVUS, OCT has become widely used in studies of plaque composition and for identification of "vulnerable" plaques prone to rupture.[14] However, the increased spatial resolution of OCT allows for evaluation of fibrous cap thickness, macrophage infiltration, and inflammation, which are beyond the scope of IVUS.[13] Optical coherence tomography is more sensitive than IVUS in identifying vessel injury and stent malapposition following PCI; however, data regarding the potential clinical benefit of OCT-guided coronary intervention are not yet available. Finally, OCT may allow for evaluation of stent strut endothelialization in vivo, an issue which is particularly important in the drug-eluting stent era.[15] However, the clinical application of OCT remains unclear until the results of current and future studies are known.

Optical Coherence Tomography Procedure

Following anticoagulant administration, the OCT catheter is advanced into the coronary artery over a wire in monorail fashion. Intracoronary nitroglycerin (50–200 μg) should be administered to promote vasodilatation prior to image acquisition and to prevent arterial spasm. Red blood cells scatter light, and therefore, OCT imaging requires a blood-free zone. This may be accomplished with saline or contrast flush, and proximal vessel occlusion in combination with continuous flushing allows for longer imaging time frames. However, proximal vessel occlusion raises concerns regarding the possibility of vessel trauma and induction of ischemia in the territory of the artery under study. Future developments in OCT technology include the use of higher speed acquisition systems that may allow imaging of an entire coronary artery in only a few seconds, without the need for proximal balloon occlusion.

Practical Pearls

- Coronary flow reserve assesses lesion significance by measuring blood flow velocity distal to the lesion. A CFR of less than 2.0 is correlated with myocardial ischemia on noninvasive testing. CFR measures the contributions of epicardial and microvascular disease.

- Fractional flow reserve assesses lesion significance by measuring pressure distal to the lesion. An FFR of less than 0.75 is correlated with myocardial ischemia on noninvasive testing, although an FFR of less than 0.80 has recently been used as the threshold to revascularize. Fractional flow reserve measures the contribution of only epicardial disease.

- Percutaneous coronary intervention may be safely deferred in patients in whom the CFR or FFR do not indicate hemodynamic significance.

- IVUS may be used to visualize the arterial lumen and the degree of vessel stenosis, as well as to characterize plaque morphology and volume. Lumen CSA of less than 3.0 mm^2 in the major epicardial vessels or less than 6.0–7.5 mm^2 in the left main coronary artery have been correlated with physiologically significant stenoses by FFR.

- IVUS guidance may improve the success of PCI by evaluating stent expansion, stent apposition, and residual stenosis, and by identifying vessel injury.

- Optical coherence tomography represents an important research tool that affords greater spatial resolution but less tissue penetration than IVUS. The clinical applications of OCT are not yet clear.

References

1. Heller LI, Cates C, Popma J, et al. Intra-coronary Doppler assessment of moderate coronary artery disease: comparison with 201Tl imaging and coronary angiography. FACTS Study Group. *Circulation.* 1997;96:484-490.

2. Serruys PW, Di Mario C, Piek J, et al. Prognostic value of intra-coronary flow velocity and diameter stenosis in assessing the short- and long-term outcomes of coronary balloon angioplasty: the DEBATE study (Doppler Endpoints Balloon Angioplasty Trial Europe). *Circulation.* 1997;96:3369-3377.

3. Pijls NH, de Bruyne B, Peels K, et al. Measurement of fractional flow reserve to assess the functional severity of coronary–artery stenoses. *N Engl J Med* 1996;334:1703-1708.

4. Claeys M, Bosmans J, Hendrix J, Vrints C. Reliability of fractional flow reserve measurements in patients with associated microvascular dysfunction: importance of flow on translesional pressure gradient. *Catheter Cardiovasc Interv.* 2001;54:427-434.

5. Chhatriwalla AK, Ragosta M, Powers ER, et al. High left ventricular mass does not limit the utility of fractional flow reserve for the physiologic assessment of lesion severity. *J Invasive Cardiol.* 2006;18:544-549.

6. Pijls NH, van Schaardenburgh P, Manoharan G, et al. Percutaneous coronary intervention of functionally nonsignificant stenosis: 5-year follow-up of the DEFER Study. *J Am Coll Cardiol.* 2007;49:2105-2111.

7. Tonino PA, De Bruyne B, Pijls NH, et al. Fractional flow reserve versus angiography for guiding percutaneous coronary intervention. *N Engl J Med* 2009; 360:213-224.

8. Takagi A, Tsurumi Y, Ishii Y, et al. Clinical potential of intravascular ultrasound for physiological assessment of coronary stenosis: relationship between quantitative ultrasound tomography and pressure-derived fractional flow reserve. *Circulation.* 1999;100:250-255.

9. Das P, Meredith I. Role of intravascular ultrasound in unprotected left main coronary intervention. *Expert Rev Cardiovasc Ther.* 2007;5:81-89.

10. Yamagishi M, Terashima M, Awano K, et al. Morphology of vulnerable coronary plaque: insights from follow-up of patients examined by intravascular ultrasound before an acute coronary syndrome. *J Am Coll Cardiol.* Jan 2000;35:106-111.

11. de Jaegere P, Mudra H, Figulla H, et al. for the MUSIC Study Investigators. Intravascular ultrasound-guided optimized stent deployment. Immediate and 6 months clinical and angiographic results from the Multicenter Ultrasound Stenting in Coronaries Study (MUSIC study). *Eur Heart J.* 1998;19:1214-1223.

12. Fitzgerald PJ, Oshima A, Hayase M, et al. Final results of the Can Routine Ultrasound Influence Stent Expansion (CRUISE) study? *Circulation.* 2000;102: 23-530.

13. Raffel OC, Akasaka T, Jang I-K. Cardiac optical coherence tomography. *Heart.* 2008;94:1200-1210.

14. Kubo T, Imanishi T, Takarada S, et al. Assessment of culprit lesion morphology in acute myocardial infarction: ability of optical coherence tomography compared with intravascular ultrasound and coronary angioscopy. *J Am Coll Cardiol.* 2007;50:933-939.

15. Takano M, Inami S, Jang IK, et al. Evaluation by optical coherence tomography of neointimal coverage of sirolimus-eluting stent three months after implantation. *Am J Cardiol.* 2007;99:1033-1038.

Chapter 7

Special Settings/ Subsets

Chapter 7a

ST-elevation Myocardial Infarction (STEMI)

Khurram Ahmad and Pranab Das

ST-elevation myocardial infarction (STEMI) is a medical emergency in which total or near total occlusion of an epicardial coronary artery ensues from a thrombus, and the myocardium supplied by this artery is at risk of necrosis and cell death. It is estimated that approximately 500,000 STEMI events per year occur in the United States.[1] Differential diagnosis for STEMI includes aortic dissection, pulmonary embolus, perforating peptic ulcer, tension pneumothorax, and Boerhaave syndrome (esophageal rupture with mediastinitis). Acute STEMI usually results from underlying atherothrombosis. Following atherosclerotic plaque disruption, the appearance occurs of substances that promote platelet activation, adhesion, aggregation, thrombin generation, and, ultimately, thrombus formation.[2] The resultant thrombus can then completely occlude the epicardial infarct artery. A wave front of myocardial necrosis begins within 15 minutes and spreads from the endocardium toward the epicardium in the absence of sufficient collateral blood supply. Angiographic evidence of coronary thrombus formation may be seen in more than 90% of patients with STEMI.

Management

Risk Assessment
The TIMI (Fig. 7a.1) is a clinical risk score with 10 baseline variables that predict 30-day mortality at presentation of patients with STEMI. Score ranges from 0 to 8. Mortality is less than 1% with a score of 0, increasing to 26% with a TIMI score of 8.[3]

Patient Selection
Primary Percutaneous Coronary Intervention
Primary percutaneous coronary intervention (PPCI) is the preferred treatment for patients with STEMI, if it (a) can be delivered in a timely fashion with door to balloon time of 90 minutes (from the initial medical contact to first balloon inflation in the catheterization laboratory), (b) by a skilled interventional

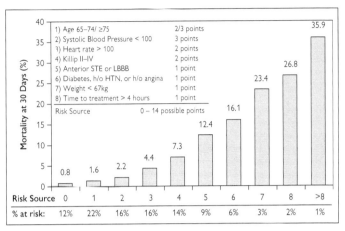

Figure 7a.1 TIMI risk score for ST elevation myocardial infarction (STEMI) for predicting 30-day mortality. From Morrow DA. TIMI risk score for ST-elevation myocardial infarction: a convenient, bedside, clinical score for risk assessment at presentation: an intravenous nPA for Treatment of Infarcting Myocardium Early II Trial Substudy. *Circulation*. 2000;102:2031-2037, with permission of the publisher (Wolters Kluwer Heart).

cardiologist (individuals who perform >75 PCI procedures per year), and (c) by a cardiac catheterization laboratory team (performs >200 PCI procedures per year, of which at least 36 are primary PCI for STEMI) with surgical backup.[4]

Rescue Percutaneous Coronary Intervention

Rescue PCI is indicated for those who fail initial fibrinolysis. Reperfusion failure after fibrinolytic therapy is suggested by a less than 50% ST elevation resolution in the lead showing the greatest degree of ST-segment elevation at presentation 90 minutes after initiation of fibrinolytic therapy and/or persistent chest pain. Rescue PCI (PCI following failed thrombolysis) has been associated with a trend toward reduced mortality, reinfarction, and heart failure.[5] Regardless of the mode of reperfusion, the most important goal is to minimize total ischemic time.[6]

Pharmacology

Table 7a.1 summarizes the pharmacology used to treat STEMI. Patients with STEMI should receive:

- Aspirin immediately
- Clopidogrel (600 mg orally) immediately as the loading dose
- Antithrombotic therapy (unfractionated heparin, low-molecular-weight heparin, fondaparinux, or bivalirudin)
- Glycoprotein IIb/IIIa inhibitors
- Primary PCI or fibrinolytic therapy for revascularization

Table 7a.1 Dosage and duration of antithrombotic therapy for management of ST elevation myocardial infarction

	Unfractionated Heparin (UFH)	Enoxaparin	Fondaparinux	Bivalirudin
Dose	Initial intravenous bolus 60 U/kg followed by an intravenous infusion of 12 U/kg/hr to keep partial thromboplastin time at 1.5–2.0 times control (approximately 50–70 seconds)	*For Cr <2.5 mg/dl in men and <2.0 mg/dl in women):* **Patient age <75:** Initial 30 mg IV bolus, followed 15 minutes later by subcutaneous injections of 1.0 mg/kg every 12 hours. **Patient age >75:** No Initial bolus. Subcutaneous dose of 0.75 mg/kg every 12 hours *For CrCl <30 mL/min,* regardless of age, the subcutaneous regimen is 1.0 mg/kg every 24 hours	Fondaparinux (creatinine is less than 3.0 mg/dL): initial dose 2.5 mg intravenously; subsequently subcutaneous injections of 2.5 mg once daily	Bivalirudin as an intravenous bolus of 0.75 mg/kg, followed by an infusion of 1.75 mg/kg/hr
Duration of therapy	No benefit of UFH beyond 48 hours in the absence of ongoing indications for anticoagulation. More prolonged UFH infusions increase the risk of development of heparin-induced thrombocytopenia.	Maintenance dosing with enoxaparin should be continued for the duration of the index hospitalization, up to 8 days.	Maintenance dosing with fondaparinux should be continued for the duration of the index hospitalization, up to 8 days.	Discontinued after the PCI
With prior treatment	For prior treatment with UFH, additional boluses of UFH as needed to support the procedure, taking into account whether GP IIb/IIIa receptor antagonists have been administered. Bivalirudin may also be used in patients treated previously with UFH.	For prior treatment with enoxaparin, if the last subcutaneous dose was administered within the prior 8 hours, no additional enoxaparin should be given; if the last subcutaneous dose was administered at least 8 to 12 hours earlier, an intravenous dose of 0.3 mg/kg of enoxaparin should be given.	For prior treatment with fondaparinux, administer additional intravenous treatment with an anticoagulant possessing anti-IIa activity taking into account whether GP IIb/IIIa receptor antagonists have been administered. Because of the risk of catheter thrombosis, fondaparinux should not be used as the sole anticoagulant to support PCI. An additional anticoagulant with anti-IIa activity should be administered.	Usually used during PCI. Bivalirudin may also be used in patients treated previously with UFH.

UFH, unfractionated heparin.

Guide Catheter Selection

Correct guide catheter selection is the key to a successful and expedient intervention. An ideal guide catheter should be able to provide the adequate support to facilitate delivery of balloon, adjunctive devices, and stents to the site of lesion. Usually, Judkins left (JL4) or extra back-up (XB) guides are used for left coronary artery interventions. An XB guide is the workhorse guide in our laboratory for left coronary interventions as it gives adequate support for both left anterior descending artery and circumflex artery interventions. Occasionally, the Amplatz left catheter may be indicated for patients who need extra guide support in situations such as distal or tortuous lesions, calcified lesions, and in acute take-off of the vessels needing intervention. The Judkins right (JR4) is the workhorse guide for right coronary artery interventions. A JR4 or hockey stick guide is preferred for interventions on vein grafts to the left coronary systems, and a JR4 or multipurpose guide is used for interventions on vein grafts to right coronary systems. Although most laboratories use 6 Fr guide catheters for intervention, use of 7 or 8 Fr guides are sometimes needed if the culprit lesions involve bifurcation stenting or use of thrombectomy.

Guidewire Choice

The choice of guidewire is entirely dependent on the preference of the operator. A wire with moderate support and high torquability is very desirable when crossing a very tight lesion. In general, a wire such as a balanced middleweight wire (BMW wire) or an ASAHI soft wire (ASAHI Light) is preferred by most operators. In acute lesion intervention, as most of the lesions are soft and distal runoff vessels are yet to be defined initially, use of hydrophilic wires are not advisable as they may easily lead to wire perforations. Hydrophilic wires are useful for access into a side branch lesion, as encountered in bifurcation stenting. Extra support wires (BHW, ASAHI Standard) are used for interventions on calcific or tortuous lesions.

Adjunctive Thrombectomy

Patients with STEMI are associated with large thrombus burden, and angiographically visible thrombus portends adverse outcomes for these patients. Rheolytic thrombectomy using Angiojet was compared in a randomized trial with conventional intervention without thrombectomy among patients undergoing primary angioplasty for acute MI (the AIMI study). There were no benefits in terms of reduced infarct size or in thrombolysis in MI (TIMI) flow, and this technique had an increased risk of major adverse cardiac events.[7] Conversely, use of aspiration thrombectomy as an adjunct to PPCI among STEMI patients showed improved myocardial blush and resolution of ST segments compared to conventional PCI without thrombus aspiration at 30 days.[8] Extended follow-up to 1 year demonstrated that this strategy reduces death and MI as well. Aspiration thrombectomy is a useful adjunctive procedure in patients with STEMI and is encouraged.

Thrombectomy devices in current use are categorized as aspiration, fragmentation, or rheolytic. Aspiration thrombectomy catheters (Export, Pronto, Fetch catheters) can be used with a 6 Fr system, and are very quick and easy to use, needing no separate preparation time. These devices aspirate thrombus manually by applying negative suction. Rheolytic thrombectomy involves a high-velocity jet of saline solution to create a Venturi effect, and the thrombi are sucked into the catheter tip. Upsizing of the sheath and temporary transvenous pacemakers are usually needed for use of Angiojet devices. Fragmentation thrombectomy employs the fragmentation technique: This uses an 8 Fr catheter with an enclosed impeller driven at 150,000 rpm by an air turbine. The rapid spinning of the impeller creates a vortex that agitates the thrombus and drags it toward the tip, where it is broken down into particles of approximately 13 μm. Figure 7a.2 shows some commonly used thrombectomy catheters.

Stent Selection: Bare Metal Versus Drug-eluting

Drug-eluting stents (DESs) have heralded a new era in interventional cardiology. In a large randomized trial comparing sirolimus-eluting stents (SESs) with bare metal stents (BMSs) in STEMI patients, SES use was associated with reduction in target vessel failure (TVF) at 1 year as compared with BMSs.[9] However, use of paclitaxel-eluting stent as compared with BMS was not associated with

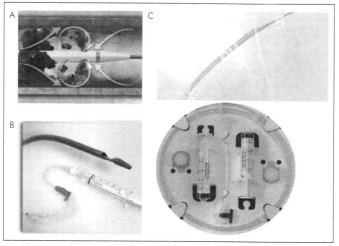

Figure 7a.2 Thrombectomy devices. (A) Different thrombectomy devices currently used in ST elevation myocardial infarction (STEMI) intervention. AngioJet thrombectomy device. (B) Different thrombectomy devices currently used in ST elevation myocardial infarction (STEMI) intervention. Pronto extraction catheter. (C) Different thrombectomy devices currently used in ST elevation myocardial infarction (STEMI) intervention. Export manual aspiration catheter.

difference in death or target lesion revascularization (TLR) at 1 year.[10] Brar et al., in their recent meta-analysis, addressed this important topic and showed that among patients with STEMI, DESs appeared to be safe, efficacious, and caused less TVR compared to BMSs, without an increase in death, MI, or stent thrombosis at 2 years.[11] However, DESs are not currently approved for use in STEMI patients due to concerns for stent thrombosis, and BMSs remain a reasonable choice in patients with STEMI (Figs. 7a.3–7a.5).

STEMI and Cardiogenic Shock

In patients with cardiogenic shock (especially those <75 years of age), severe congestive heart failure/pulmonary edema, or hemodynamically compromising ventricular arrhythmias (regardless of age), coronary angiography with intent to perform PCI is preferred to fibrinolytic treatment, provided further invasive management is not considered futile or unsuitable given the clinical circumstances.[12] Current American College of Cardiology/American Heart Association (ACC/AHA) guidelines list the intra-aortic balloon pump (IABP) as a class IB recommendation in patients with STEMI and shock, when shock cannot be quickly reversed by pharmacologic therapy. Use of percutaneous circulatory-assist devices (e.g., Impella device) may also be of use for patients with cardiogenic shock and is discussed in Chapter 7b.

Conclusion

The primary goal in STEMI is to salvage maximum myocardium at the earliest possible time. With early presentation (<3 hours) and a potential delay to invasive strategy, fibrinolysis may be the preferred modality for reperfusion. Primary percutaneous coronary intervention is usually preferred for all patients when it can be provided by skilled personnel in a timely manner (door to balloon time <90 minutes). Primary percutaneous coronary intervention is also preferred for patients with high-risk presentations (cardiogenic shock, electrical instability, or congestive heart failure) and for patients older than age 75. Emerging data suggest that DES superior to BMSs among STEMI patients, but DESs not approved for STEMI use at this time.

Practical Pearls

- Use of front-loaded clopidogrel in addition to aspirin in the emergency department may help improve outcomes in STEMI.

- One should make a point to always look at any previous available angiograms and also know the graft anatomy whenever possible before embarking on a STEMI intervention.

- Using a diagnostic catheter for the non-culprit artery and then proceeding with the guide directly for the culprit artery saves time and muscle during STEMI intervention.

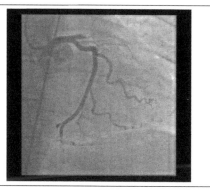

Figure 7a.3 Acute anterior ST elevation MI (STEMI) from thrombotic occlusion of large left anterior descending artery.

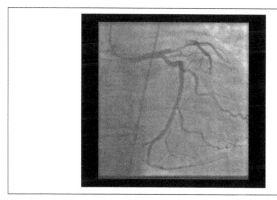

Figure 7a.4 Visible thrombus with TIMI I flow in left anterior descending artery following initial balloon inflation.

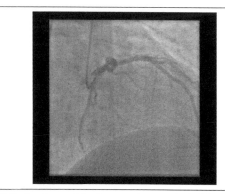

Figure 7a.5 Final angiogram following stent placement in the left anterior descending artery.

- Intervention performed only on the culprit artery and staged intervention of other critical stenoses is the recommended strategy to ensure good outcomes.
- Straight anteroposterior (AP) or left anterior oblique (LAO) are the best views to engage left coronary guides; left anterior oblique 30 degrees is the best view for right coronary engagement. Right anterior oblique (RAO) caudal or LAO caudal views are the best to wire a lesion in the proximal left anterior descending artery (LAD) and proximal or distal circumflex artery (Cx). LAO or RAO cranial views are best suited for wiring lesions in the mid to distal LAD.
- Positioning of a stent in the proximal LAD or circumflex should always be done after confirming the proximal extent of the stent in one of the caudal views to avoid extension into the left main artery.
- A slight bend at the tip of the guidewire is sufficient for accessing the left anterior descending artery. A sharper or more acute bend or double bends are needed to access the circumflex artery.
- Use of smaller balloons, such as 2 mm × 15 mm or 2.5 mm × 15 mm, are preferable for predilatation as they have a smaller and easier crossing profile, which helps to adequately dilate the lesion to establish some flow and thus allow visualization of the distal vessels.
- Liberal use of IABP among high-risk patients may improve procedure outcomes.
- Knowledge of patient's socioeconomic status, insurance status, medication and clinical compliance, and family support are useful when deciding what type of stents to choose for a particular patient. This helps minimize stent thrombosis from medication noncompliance if a DES is used.
- Aspiration thrombectomy followed by direct stenting during PPCI appears to be the optimal strategy in improving short- and long-term outcomes.

References

1. American Heart Association. *Heart disease and stroke statistics-2004 update.* Dallas, TX: American Heart Association, 2003.

2. Davies MJ, Woolf N, Robertson WB. Pathology of acute myocardial infarction with particular reference to occlusive coronary thrombi. *Br Heart J.* 1976;38: 659-664.

3. Morrow DA, Antman EM, Charlesworth A, et al. TIMI risk score for ST-elevation myocardial infarction: a convenient, bedside, clinical score for risk assessment at presentation: an intravenous nPA for treatment of infarcting myocardium early II trial substudy. *Circulation.* 2000;102:2031-2037.

4. Antman EM, Anbe DT, Armstrong PW, et al. ACC/AHA guidelines for the management of patients with ST-elevation myocardial infarction – Executive summary: a report of the American College of Cardiology/American Heart Association Task Force on Practice Guidelines (Writing Committee to Revise the 1999 Guidelines for the Management of Patients with Acute Myocardial Infarction). *Circulation.* 2004;110:588-636.

5. Wijeysundera HC, Vijayaraghavan R, Nallamothu BK, et al. Rescue angioplasty or repeat fibrinolysis after failed fibrinolytic therapy for ST-segment myocardial infarction: a meta-analysis of randomized trials. *J Am Coll Cardiol.* 2007;49:422-430.

6. Bradley EH, Herrin J, Wang Y, et al. Strategies for reducing the door-to-balloon time in acute myocardial infarction *N Engl J Med.* 2006;355:2308-2320.

7. Ali A, Cox D, Dib N, et al.; for the AIMI Investigator. The AiMI Trial. AngioJet in Acute Myocardial Infarction Trial. *J Am Coll Cardiol.* 2006;48:244–252.

8. Svilaas T, Vlaar PJ, van der Horst IC, et al. Thrombus aspiration during primary percutaneous coronary intervention. *N Engl J Med.* 2008;358:557-567.

9. Spaulding C, Henry P, Teiger E, et al. Sirolimus eluting versus uncoated stents in acute myocardial infarction. *N Engl J Med.* 2006;355:1093-1104.

10. Laarman GJ, Suttorp MJ, Dirksen MT, et al. Paclitaxel-eluting versus uncoated stents in primary percutaneous coronary intervention. *N Engl J Med.* 2006;355:1105-1113.

11. Brar SS, Leon MB, Stone GW, et al. Use of drug-eluting stents in acute myocardial infarction: a systematic review and meta-analysis. *J Am Coll Cardiol.* 2009;53:1677-1689.

12. Antman EM, Hand M, Bates ER, et al. 2007 focused update of the ACC/AHA 2004 guidelines for the management of patients with ST-elevation myocardial infarction. *Circulation.* 2008;117:296-329.

Chapter 7b

Percutaneous Interventions in Cardiogenic Shock

Amer K. Ardati and Hitinder S. Gurm

Cardiogenic shock (CS) remains a high-risk clinical condition, with a mortality rate approaching 66% despite aggressive invasive therapy.[1] This clinical syndrome of reduced cardiac output with elevated or normal filling pressures resulting in end-organ hypoperfusion may have a myriad of etiologies. Appropriate therapy should focus on reversing the cause of shock and providing adequate support until recovery or definitive therapy is delivered. Percutaneous therapeutic options are divided into revascularization and mechanical hemodynamic support.

Patient Management

The initial evaluation of patients with CS should focus on identifying the etiology of shock. Generally, CS is divided into shock secondary to cardiac ischemia in the setting of acute coronary syndromes (ACS) and shock unrelated to ischemia. Shock due to ACS may be caused by loss of ventricular systolic function or by a mechanical complication of the infarction, such as acute mitral regurgitation, ventricular septal defect, ventricular free-wall rupture, or tamponade. Nonischemic shock may be caused by loss of volume control in patients with chronic heart failure, sudden adrenergic surge, arrhythmia, or myocarditis. The history and physical examination should focus on the following elements:

- Presence of acute coronary syndrome and time of symptom onset
- History of preexisting heart failure
- Degree of end-organ involvement (e.g., mental status changes, respiratory failure, oliguria, hepatopathy, metabolic acidosis, or digital ischemia)
- Vital signs, heart rhythm, lung sounds, murmurs, pulsus paradoxus, or Kussmaul's sign

The patient should be evaluated in an intensive care setting, such as the emergency department, intensive care unit (ICU), or angiography suite. Initial testing should include:

- 12-Lead electrocardiogram (EKG) and continuous telemetry
- Oxygen saturation

- Arterial blood gases (ABGs) with serum lactate
- Basic chemistry, including serum sodium, potassium, and bicarbonate levels
- Complete blood count (CBC)
- Prothrombin time
- Portable chest x-ray

If the patient is found to be in respiratory failure, emergent endotracheal intubation and mechanical ventilation should be started. Life-threatening arrhythmia should be treated following the Adult Cardiac Life Support protocol. If a mechanical complication is suspected, immediate echocardiography should be performed. At this point, the patient's management will depend on whether an ACS event is occurring.

Cardiogenic Shock Associated with Acute Coronary Syndrome

Patients with evidence of ACS should be sent for emergent cardiac catheterization, with the goal of revascularization and mechanical support. Current American College of Cardiology/American Heart Association (ACC/AHA) guidelines suggest that the first step in the invasive management of CS secondary to ACS is to place an intra-aortic balloon pump (IABP).

Intra-aortic Balloon Pump

Placement of an IABP is a Class I indication in patients with CS related to ST elevation myocardial infarction (STEMI) and is a IIa recommendation in patients with non-ST elevation MI/unstable angina (NSTEMI/UA).[2,3] Initial evidence supporting the benefit of IABP for CS in the setting of acute MI (AMI) was extracted from retrospective data analysis that suggested improved survival to discharge and 1-year survival.[4,5] The observed mortality benefit of IABP appears to have been driven by AMI patients treated with thrombolytics, in whom IABP use coincided with an increase in revascularization procedures.[6,7] Small randomized studies have not been adequately designed to establish the mortality benefit of IABP in CS secondary to AMI.[8,9] Nonetheless, it appears that patients with CS secondary to AMI tend to have better outcomes when treated with IABP support in centers with high IABP use, regardless of method of revascularization.[10] A contemporary review of IABP outcomes suggests that complications occur in 8.1% of patients who receive IABP. Major events such as limb ischemia, bleeding, balloon leak, or death related to IABP only occurred in 2.7% of cases.[11] Contraindications to IABP include moderate to severe aortic valve insufficiency, abdominal aortic aneurysm, uncontrolled bleeding or sepsis, and bilateral severe peripheral arterial disease.[12]

Technique

- *Equipment selection*: Intra-aortic balloon pumps are produced by multiple manufacturers and are available in different sizes. The patient's height and body surface area dictate the volume and sheath size of the balloon used.

- *Access*: To facilitate coronary angiography and PCI, it is helpful to insert the IABP via the left common femoral artery. In the presence of severe bilateral peripheral arterial disease, an IABP may be placed with surgical assistance via an axillary artery cut-down. Note that the IABP may be placed with or without an introducer sheath. If sheathless insertion is required, the tear-away introducer sheath should be removed after the device is positioned.

- *Positioning*: Once access is obtained, the balloon tip should be positioned distal to the take-off of the left subclavian artery. A helpful landmark is the inferior border of the left clavicle.

- *Pump initiation*: The timing of inflation and deflation can be triggered by EKG information, systemic arterial pressure wave forms, or may be preset by the operator, as in the case of ventricular fibrillation or cardiopulmonary bypass. Appropriate timing of balloon inflation and deflation is needed to achieve optimal IABP support (Fig. 7b.1). Fluoroscopic evaluation of the entire length of the balloon should be performed to ensure adequate balloon inflation and position.

- *Postinsertion care*: The insertion sheath and balloon catheter should be sutured to the patient. Clear sterile dressing should be placed over the insertion site. The patient must remain supine as long as the IABP is in place. Although standard practice has been to provide systemic anticoagulation with heparin during IABP use, no randomized studies have demonstrated a benefit to this strategy. A single-center randomized trial of 153 patients treated with IABP found no benefit to systemic anticoagulation with heparin and an increase in bleeding outcomes.[13]

- *Removal*: Once IABP use is no longer required and removal is desired, systemic anticoagulation should be withheld. Standard sheath removal precautions should be taken to manage pain and vasovagal reactions. The insertion site should be allowed to back bleed momentarily to eject any possible clot. Hemostatic pressure should be maintained for a minimum of 30 minutes. Once hemostasis is achieved, the patient should remain supine for 6 hours.

Percutaneous Coronary Intervention

Once hemodynamic control is obtained, focus should quickly to turn to achieving revascularization. The advent of emergent reperfusion therapy in AMI has altered the incidence of CS worldwide.[14–17] Immediate revascularization has been shown to improve both short- and long-term outcomes in patients who suffer CS secondary to AMI.[18,19] Observational studies initially suggested that revascularization in CS reduced 30-day mortality by 22%–33%, but these reports were hampered by selection bias.[20,21] Randomized trial data supporting PCI in CS come from the Should We Emergently Revascularize Occluded Coronaries for Cardiogenic Shock (SHOCK) trial, which randomized 302 patients with CS due to LV dysfunction in the setting of AMI to medical therapy or emergent revascularization. All patients were recommended treatment with IABP. Medical patients were given thrombolytics if appropriate and advised to delay revascularization by a minimum of 54 hours after randomization. Patients assigned to early revascularization were advised to have either coronary artery

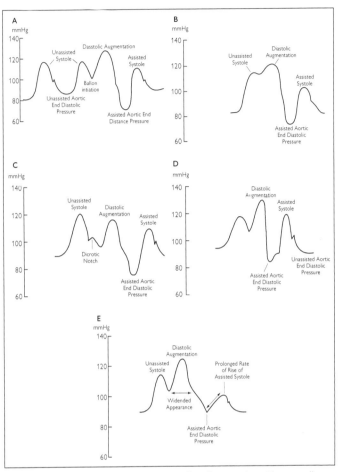

Figure 7b.1 (A) Systemic arterial pressure waveform from a patient with a normally functioning intra-aortic balloon pump (IABP) device, in whom the IABP device is programmed to inflate during every other cardiac cycle (commonly referred to as "1:2," or one inflation for every two cardiac cycles). With the first beat, aortic systolic and end-diastolic pressures are shown without IABP support and are therefore unassisted. With the second beat, the balloon inflates with the appearance of the dicrotic notch, and peak-augmented diastolic pressure is inscribed. With balloon deflation, assisted end-diastolic pressure and assisted systolic pressure are observed. To confirm that the IABP is producing maximal hemodynamic benefit, the peak diastolic augmentation should be greater than the unassisted systolic pressure, and the two assisted pressures should be less than the unassisted values. (B) Systemic arterial pressure waveform from a subject in whom balloon inflation occurs too early, before aortic valve closure. Consequently, the left ventricle is forced to empty against an inflated balloon; the corresponding increase in afterload may increase myocardial oxygen demands and worsen systolic function. (C) Systemic arterial pressure waveform from a patient in whom balloon inflation occurs too late, well after the beginning of diastole, thereby minimizing diastolic pressure

bypass graft (CABG) surgery or PCI as soon as possible within 6 hours of randomization. Patients assigned to early revascularization had decreased mortality at 30 days, 6 months, 3 years, and 6 years (absolute risk reduction: 9.3%, 12.8%, 13.1%, and 13.1%, respectively).

Technique

- *Equipment selection*: Standard diagnostic angiography and intervention equipment should be prepared. In the setting of AMI, consideration of catheter thrombectomy should be made. A pulmonary artery catheter equipped with a catheter cover (e.g., "swan saver" or "swan-dom") should be prepared as well.

- *Access*: A 6 Fr arterial access should be sufficient in a majority of cases. An 8 Fr venous access sheath should also be placed to facilitate delivery of vasopressors, inotropes, and pulmonary artery catheterization. It is recommended that the IABP be placed on standby mode when advancing catheters in the aorta. Intra-aortic balloon pumping should resume once the coronary catheter has reached the ascending aorta.

- *Anticoagulation*: The current standard of care for anticoagulation during ACS complicated by CS is heparin and glycoprotein IIb/IIIa inhibition. A retrospective study of 89 patients with AMI complicated by CS treated with bivalirudin and provisional glycoprotein IIb/IIIa inhibition suggests that a bivalirudin-based strategy may be safe and effective.[22] Anticoagulation should not be given if ventricular free-wall rupture is detected.

- *Lesion selection*: The infarct-related artery should be identified promptly and revascularized first. No clear data exist to address the risks and benefits of multivessel PCI in CS. In the SHOCK trial, single-stage multivessel PCI was performed in nearly 14% of patients and was associated with a 35% reduction in 1-year survival.[23,24] It is difficult to make conclusions based on this observation, due to the inherent selection bias involved with this subset of patients. Current recommendations suggest that if CS persists despite revascularization of the infarct-related artery, other potential PCI targets should be treated. In the presence of severe three-vessel coronary disease or left main coronary disease, the patient should be referred for emergent bypass surgery. In the SHOCK trial, patients who received bypass had similar outcomes to those who received PCI.[23]

---

augmentation. (D) Systemic arterial pressure waveform from a patient in whom balloon deflation occurs too early, before the end of diastole. This may shorten the period of diastolic pressure augmentation. A corresponding transient decrease in aortic pressure may promote retrograde arterial flow from the carotid or coronary arteries, possibly inducing cerebral or myocardial ischemia. (E) Systemic arterial pressure waveform from a subject in whom balloon deflation occurs too late, after the end of diastole, thereby producing the same deleterious consequences as early balloon inflation (increased left ventricular afterload, with a resultant increase in myocardial oxygen demands and a worsening of systolic function). Reprinted from Trost JC, Hillis LD. Intra-aortic balloon counterpulsation. *Am J Cardiol.* 2006; 97:1391-1398, with permission of the publisher (Elsevier).

- *Device selection*: The presence of a mechanical complication such as acute mitral regurgitation or ventricular septal defect may require surgery in the short term. Alternatively, severe left ventricular (LV) systolic dysfunction and continued shock may trigger the need for transplant or permanent LV assist device placement. If a surgical intervention is anticipated, placement of a stent should be avoided and reperfusion should be performed with angioplasty only.

Special Consideration

- *Delayed presentation*: The current ACC/AHA guidelines for the management of AMI emphasize urgent revascularization for patients who present within 12 hours of symptom onset. In patients with CS, the window of opportunity is prolonged to 36 hours after the index MI as long as revascularization is performed within 18 hours of the onset of shock (Class Ia for patients <75 years old, IIa for patients ≥75).[2]

- *Non-ST elevation myocardial infarction (NSTEMI)*: Nearly 2% of NSTEMI patients will develop CS; moreover, NSTEMI patients represent 17%–30% of all CS patients.[25,26] Patients with NSTEMI complicated by CS tend to be older, have renal insufficiency, have more advanced coronary disease, and develop shock later than their STEMI counterparts. Patients with NSTEMI and CS have similar 30-day mortality to those with STEMI and CS. Current ACC/AHA guidelines recommend early invasive management of all NSTEMI patients within 48 hours of presentation, based on data from multiple clinical trials showing a reduction in mortality and nonfatal MI and recurrent UA.[3,27] All early invasive clinical trials in NSTEMI have excluded patients with CS. Given the high mortality of CS, the benefits of emergent revascularization in NSTEMI CS are inferred from the STEMI population.

- *Elderly*: Patients 75 years and older only accounted for 18% of SHOCK trial participants. In this small subset, early revascularization did not appear to offer a mortality benefit. The small sample size and the heterogeneity in baseline characteristics of the patients (particularity lower ejection fraction in patients randomized to early revascularization) may have contributed to the absence of a beneficial effect.[28] Subsequent registry analysis suggests that elderly patients do in fact have a mortality benefit from early revascularization commensurate with results seen in younger patients.[29]

- *Absence of primary PCI*: If the patient presents to a facility without PCI capability, fibrinolytics should be given if (1) time to PCI is greater than 90 minutes, (2) STEMI onset occurred less than 3 hour ago, and (3) there is an absence of contraindications to fibrinolytic therapy. Once fibrinolysis is started, the patient should be transferred to a PCI center immediately in case mechanical support is required.

Cardiogenic Shock without Ischemia

Patients with CS unrelated to ischemia are at high risk of death and require comprehensive critical care to prevent poor outcomes. As previously mentioned, the etiology of shock must be determined and reversed. The patient should be cared for in an ICU setting. If medical management fails to quickly relieve shock, invasive hemodynamic support must be considered. The most widely available and simplest form of mechanical support is the IABP. Should a patient fail IABP support or appear to have biventricular heart failure, concomitant lung injury, or severe LV systolic dysfunction, several alternative percutaneous assist strategies exist.

Extracorporeal Membrane Oxygenation

Extracorporeal membrane oxygenation (ECMO) offers total cardiopulmonary support via peripherally placed arterial and venous access points. Access is typically achieved with 15 Fr catheters in the femoral artery and vein. The removal of venous blood and external oxygenation allows for biventricular support in cases where recovery is expected or definitive therapy is planned. Thirty-day survival for patients with CS who require ECMO has been reported as high as 38%.[30] Initiating ECMO during cardiopulmonary resuscitation (CPR) has worse outcomes than starting support before complete hemodynamic collapse occurs. Patients with myocarditis tend to have higher survival rates than other ECMO recipients.[31] A study assessing the utility of ECMO in temporizing high-risk CS patients (systolic blood pressure ≤75 mm Hg despite two inotropes with or without IABP, multiorgan failure, and mechanical ventilation) prior to left ventricular assist device placement (LVAD) found that patients who were able to survive ECMO had 1-year outcomes similar to those of lower-risk patients who proceeded directly to LVAD placement.[32] Complications related to ECMO use include access site bleeding; thrombotic complications, including stroke and ischemic limbs; infection; and left ventricular distention.

Impella Device

The Impella 2.5 device (Abiomed, Danvers, MA) is an axial flow pump inserted percutaneously via a 13 Fr introducer into the femoral artery. The device is placed across the aortic valve, draws blood from the left ventricle, and pumps it into the ascending aorta at a maximum rate of 2.5 L/min (Fig. 7b.2).

Insertion and continued support requires anticoagulation with heparin to reach an ACT of 160–180 sec.[33] A small study that randomized 26 patients with CS secondary to AMI to Impella versus IABP support showed that the Impella tended to produce higher cardiac output and mean arterial pressures than that seen in IABP-treated patients. Impella patients tended to have more blood transfusions, and device insertion took 8 minutes longer than IABP deployment.[34] In addition to improving cardiac output and systemic blood pressure, Impella use has been shown to improve coronary perfusion pressure and improve coronary flow reserve.[35] Complications of Impella use include hemolysis, stroke, ventricular arrhythmia, and bleeding.

TandemHeart

The TandemHeart (CardiacAssist, Pittsburgh, PA) is an extracorporeal centrifugal pump that aspirates blood from the left atrium and returns it to the arterial circulation via a 15 Fr femoral artery catheter. Left atrial access is achieved with

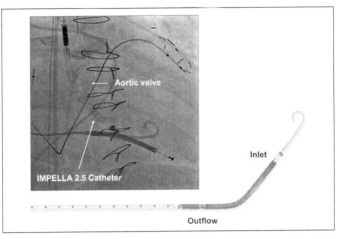

Figure 7b.2 The Impella 2.5 catheter positioned across the aortic valve. Reprinted from Dixon SR et al. A prospective feasibility trial investigating the use of the Impella 2.5 system in patients undergoing high-risk percutaneous coronary intervention (The PROTECT I Trial): initial U.S. experience. *JACC: Cardiovasc Interv.* 2009;2(41):91-96, with permission of the publisher (Elsevier).

a 21 Fr catheter introduced into the femoral vein and then across the interatrial septum under fluoroscopic guidance. The device can achieve an output of 4.0 L/min. The TandemHeart system requires systemic anticoagulation with heparin to achieve an ACT of 400 seconds during insertion and an ACT of 200 seconds or more during support.[36] Two small randomized trials with a total of 83 patients with CS have demonstrated that TandemHeart use results in higher cardiac output, lower pulmonary capillary wedge pressure, and higher systemic blood pressure than IABP therapy.[37,38] The TandemHeart device has also been used to treat CS secondary to right ventricular failure in the setting of inferior MI. To provide right ventricular support, the inflow catheter is positioned in the right atrium, and the outflow catheter is placed in the main pulmonary artery.[39] Complications of TandemHeart use include atrial rupture during insertion, hemolysis, stroke, and bleeding (see Table 7b.1).

Conclusion

Cardiogenic shock is a high-risk clinical condition that requires prompt critical care. Careful and concise evaluation on presentation is necessary to identify the etiology of shock and to triage the patient to appropriate therapy including IABP[40] or Impella device.[41] The use of invasive management can improve

Table 7b.1 Comparison of different forms of percutaneous hemodynamic support for patients with cardiogenic shock

	IABP	ECMO	Impella	TandemHeart
Availability	+++++	+	+++	++
Systemic anticoagulation	–	+++	+++	+++
Minimal arterial access sheath	7F	15F	13F	15F
Special staffing and support	ICU	ICU and Perfusionist	ICU	ICU
Biventricular support	–	+++	–	– (may be used for isolated RV support)
Increased cardiac output	1 L/min	5 L/min	2.5 L/min	4 L/min
Technical difficulty	+	+	++	++++
Bedside insertion	+	+	–	–
Cost	+	+++++	+++	++++

short- and long-term outcomes. Patients with CS secondary to ACS benefit from revascularization. Mechanical support options are varied, and selection should be based on individual patient characteristics.

Practical Pearls

• Patients with CS should be divided into those with ACS and those without ischemia early on.

• Mechanical complications of ACS should be considered and managed prior to providing anticoagulation and placement of stents.

• Several mechanical support options are available, and these should be used according to the patient's needs and characteristics.

References

1. Hochman JS, Boland J, Sleeper LA, et al. Current spectrum of cardiogenic shock and effect of early revascularization on mortality. Results of an International Registry. SHOCK Registry Investigators. *Circulation*. 1995;91:873-881.

2. Antman EM, Anbe DT, Armstrong PW, et al. ACC/AHA guidelines for the management of patients with ST-elevation myocardial infarction: a report of the American College of Cardiology/American Heart Association Task Force on Practice Guidelines (Committee to Revise the 1999 Guidelines for the Management of patients with acute myocardial infarction). *J Am Coll Cardiol*. 2004;44:E1-E211.

3. Anderson JL, Adams CD, Antman EM, et al. ACC/AHA 2007 guidelines for the management of patients with unstable angina/non ST-elevation myocardial infarction: a report of the American College of Cardiology/American Heart Association Task Force on Practice Guidelines (Writing Committee to Revise the 2002 Guidelines for the Management of Patients with Unstable Angina/Non ST-Elevation Myocardial Infarction): developed in collaboration with the American College of Emergency Physicians, the Society for Cardiovascular Angiography and Interventions, and the Society of Thoracic Surgeons: endorsed by the American Association of Cardiovascular and Pulmonary Rehabilitation and the Society for Academic Emergency Medicine. *Circulation.* 2007;116:e148-304.

4. Kovack PJ, Rasak MA, Bates ER, Ohman EM, Stomel RJ. Thrombolysis plus aortic counterpulsation: improved survival in patients who present to community hospitals with cardiogenic shock. *J Am Coll Cardiol.* 1997;29:1454-1458.

5. Anderson RD, Ohman EM, Holmes DR, Jr., et al. Use of intraaortic balloon counterpulsation in patients presenting with cardiogenic shock: observations from the GUSTO-I Study. Global Utilization of Streptokinase and TPA for Occluded Coronary Arteries. *J Am Coll Cardiol.* 1997;30:708-715.

6. Barron HV, Every NR, Parsons LS, et al. The use of intra-aortic balloon counterpulsation in patients with cardiogenic shock complicating acute myocardial infarction: data from the National Registry of Myocardial Infarction 2. *Am Heart J.* 2001;141:933-939.

7. Sjauw KD, Engstrom AE, Vis MM, et al. A systematic review and meta-analysis of intra-aortic balloon pump therapy in ST-elevation myocardial infarction: should we change the guidelines? *Eur Heart J.* 2009;30:459-468.

8. Ohman EM, Nanas J, Stomel RJ, et al. Thrombolysis and counterpulsation to improve survival in myocardial infarction complicated by hypotension and suspected cardiogenic shock or heart failure: results of the TACTICS Trial. *J Thromb Thrombolysis.* 2005;19:33-39.

9. Ohman EM, George BS, White CJ, et al. Use of aortic counterpulsation to improve sustained coronary artery patency during acute myocardial infarction. Results of a randomized trial. The Randomized IABP Study Group. *Circulation.* 1994;90:792-799.

10. Chen EW, Canto JG, Parsons LS, et al. Relation between hospital intra-aortic balloon counterpulsation volume and mortality in acute myocardial infarction complicated by cardiogenic shock. *Circulation.* 2003;108:951-957.

11. Stone GW, Ohman EM, Miller MF, et al. Contemporary utilization and outcomes of intra-aortic balloon counterpulsation in acute myocardial infarction: the benchmark registry. *J Am Coll Cardiol.* 2003;41:1940-1945.

12. Baim DS, Grossman W. *Grossman's cardiac catheterization, angiography, and intervention,* 7th ed. Philadelphia: Lippincott, Williams & Wilkins, 2005.

13. Jiang CY, Zhao LL, Wang JA, Mohammod B. Anticoagulation therapy in intra-aortic balloon counterpulsation: does IABP really need anti-coagulation? *J Zhejiang Univ Sci* 2003;4:607-611.

14. Jeger RV, Radovanovic D, Hunziker PR, et al. Ten-year trends in the incidence and treatment of cardiogenic shock. *Ann Intern Med.* 2008;149:618-626.

15. Goldberg RJ, Spencer FA, Gore JM, Lessard D, Yarzebski J. Thirty-year trends (1975 to 2005) in the magnitude of, management of, and hospital death rates associated with cardiogenic shock in patients with acute myocardial infarction: a population-based perspective. *Circulation.* 2009;119:1211-1219.

16. Babaev A, Frederick PD, Pasta DJ, Every N, Sichrovsky T, Hochman JS. Trends in management and outcomes of patients with acute myocardial infarction complicated by cardiogenic shock. *JAMA*. 2005;294:448-454.

17. Fox KA, Steg PG, Eagle KA, et al. Decline in rates of death and heart failure in acute coronary syndromes, 1999-2006. *JAMA*. 2007;297:1892-1900.

18. Hochman JS, Sleeper LA, Webb JG, et al. Early revascularization in acute myocardial infarction complicated by cardiogenic shock. SHOCK Investigators. Should We Emergently Revascularize Occluded Coronaries for Cardiogenic Shock. *N Engl J Med*. 1999;341:625-634.

19. Hochman JS, Sleeper LA, Webb JG, et al. Early revascularization and long-term survival in cardiogenic shock complicating acute myocardial infarction. *JAMA*. 2006;295:2511-2515.

20. Lee L, Bates ER, Pitt B, Walton JA, Laufer N, O'Neill WW. Percutaneous transluminal coronary angioplasty improves survival in acute myocardial infarction complicated by cardiogenic shock. *Circulation*. 1988;78:1345-1351.

21. Berger PB, Holmes DR, Jr., Stebbins AL, Bates ER, Califf RM, Topol EJ. Impact of an aggressive invasive catheterization and revascularization strategy on mortality in patients with cardiogenic shock in the Global Utilization of Streptokinase and Tissue Plasminogen Activator for Occluded Coronary Arteries (GUSTO-I) trial. An observational study. *Circulation*. 1997;96:122-127.

22. Bonello L, De Labriolle A, Roy P, et al. Bivalirudin with provisional glycoprotein IIb/IIIa inhibitors in patients undergoing primary angioplasty in the setting of cardiogenic shock. *Am J Cardiol*. 2008;102:287-291.

23. White HD, Assmann SF, Sanborn TA, et al. Comparison of percutaneous coronary intervention and coronary artery bypass grafting after acute myocardial infarction complicated by cardiogenic shock: results from the Should We Emergently Revascularize Occluded Coronaries for Cardiogenic Shock (SHOCK) trial. *Circulation*. 2005;112:1992-2001.

24. Webb JG, Lowe AM, Sanborn TA, et al. Percutaneous coronary intervention for cardiogenic shock in the SHOCK trial. *J Am Coll Cardiol*. 2003;42:1380-1386.

25. Holmes DR, Jr., Berger PB, Hochman JS, et al. Cardiogenic shock in patients with acute ischemic syndromes with and without ST-segment elevation. *Circulation*. 1999;100:2067-20673.

26. Jacobs AK, French JK, Col J, et al. Cardiogenic shock with non-ST-segment elevation myocardial infarction: a report from the SHOCK Trial Registry. SHould we emergently revascularize Occluded coronaries for Cardiogenic shocK? *J Am Coll Cardiol*. 2000;36:1091-1096.

27. Bavry AA, Kumbhani DJ, Rassi AN, Bhatt DL, Askari AT. Benefit of early invasive therapy in acute coronary syndromes: a meta-analysis of contemporary randomized clinical trials. *J Am Coll Cardiol*. 2006;48:1319-1325.

28. Dzavik V, Sleeper LA, Cocke TP, et al. Early revascularization is associated with improved survival in elderly patients with acute myocardial infarction complicated by cardiogenic shock: a report from the SHOCK Trial Registry. *Eur Heart J*. 2003;24:828-837.

29. Dzavik V, Sleeper LA, Picard MH, et al. Outcome of patients aged ≥75 years in the SHould we emergently revascularize Occluded Coronaries in cardiogenic shocK (SHOCK) trial: do elderly patients with acute myocardial infarction complicated by cardiogenic shock respond differently to emergent revascularization? *Am Heart J*. 2005;149:1128-1134.

30. Smedira NG, Moazami N, Golding CM, et al. Clinical experience with 202 adults receiving extracorporeal membrane oxygenation for cardiac failure: survival at five years. *J Thorac Cardiovasc Surg.* 2001;122:92-102.

31. Combes A, Leprince P, Luyt CE, et al. Outcomes and long-term quality-of-life of patients supported by extracorporeal membrane oxygenation for refractory cardiogenic shock. *Crit Care Med.* 2008;36:1404-1411.

32. Pagani FD, Lynch W, Swaniker F, et al. Extracorporeal life support to left ventricular assist device bridge to heart transplant: a strategy to optimize survival and resource utilization. *Circulation.* 1999;100:II206-210.

33. *Impella 2.5 Circulator support system: Quick reference guide.* Danvers, MA: Abiomed, Inc, 2007.

34. Seyfarth M, Sibbing D, Bauer I, et al. A randomized clinical trial to evaluate the safety and efficacy of a percutaneous left ventricular assist device versus intra-aortic balloon pumping for treatment of cardiogenic shock caused by myocardial infarction. *J Am Coll Cardiol.* 2008;52:1584-1588.

35. Remmelink M, Sjauw KD, Henriques JP, et al. Effects of left ventricular unloading by Impella recover LP2.5 on coronary hemodynamics. *Catheter Cardiovasc Interv.* 2007;70:532-537.

36. *TandemHeart: guide to patient management.* Pittsburgh, PA: CardiacAssist, Inc, 2006.

37. Burkhoff D, Cohen H, Brunckhorst C, O'Neill WW. A randomized multicenter clinical study to evaluate the safety and efficacy of the TandemHeart percutaneous ventricular assist device versus conventional therapy with intraaortic balloon pumping for treatment of cardiogenic shock. *Am Heart J.* 2006;152:469 e1-8.

38. Thiele H, Sick P, Boudriot E, et al. Randomized comparison of intra-aortic balloon support with a percutaneous left ventricular assist device in patients with revascularized acute myocardial infarction complicated by cardiogenic shock. *Eur Heart J.* 2005;26:1276-1283.

39. Giesler GM, Gomez JS, Letsou G, Vooletich M, Smalling RW. Initial report of percutaneous right ventricular assist for right ventricular shock secondary to right ventricular infarction. *Catheter Cardiovasc Interv.* 2006;68:263-266.

40. Trost JC, Hillis LD. Intra-aortic balloon counterpulsation. *Am J Cardiol.* 2006;97:1391-1398.

41. Dixon SR, Henriques JP, Mauri L, et al. A prospective feasibility trial investigating the use of the Impella 2.5 system in patients undergoing high-risk percutaneous coronary intervention (The PROTECT I Trial): initial U.S. experience. *JACC Cardiovasc Interv.* 2009;2:91-96.

Chapter 7c

Saphenous Vein Graft Intervention

Khurram Ahmad and Pranab Das

More than 400,000 coronary artery bypass graft (CABG) operations are performed annually in the United States, with the saphenous vein graft (SVG) as the major type of conduit. Only about 80% of SVGs may remain patent 5 years after surgery, and about 60% are patent at 7–10 years. Disease in the SVG involves three discrete processes: thrombosis, intimal hyperplasia, and atherosclerosis. During the first month after bypass surgery, vein graft obstruction results from thrombotic occlusion. Intimal hyperplasia is the major disease process in venous grafts between 1 month and 1 year after implantation. Beyond the first year after bypass surgery, atherosclerosis is the dominant process causing the attrition of saphenous veins.[1] Repeat CABG or percutaneous coronary intervention (PCI) is needed for nearly 5% at 5 years and 20% at 10 years.[2] The success of PCI of SVG ranges from 70% to 90%, based on the degree of stenosis. Degenerated SVGs, aorto-ostial lesions, and older grafts are associated with lower success during PCI.[3]

Proximal Anastomoses of the Venous Grafts

It is helpful to review the operative report or previous angiogram to help minimize the amount of dye during cannulation of vein grafts. Surgical clips left after bypass surgery also help in localizing the grafts. In the absence of clips, a general knowledge of the graft location may help. Grafts to the left coronary artery arise from the left anterior surface of aorta. Grafts to the circumflex are usually placed higher than grafts to left anterior descending (LAD) artery. Grafts to the right coronary artery are commonly anastomosed superior to the native right coronary ostium. A 30-degree left anterior oblique (LAO) aortogram may also help in localizing the graft anastomoses. Grafts to the left coronary artery (LCA) are best cannulated in a right anterior oblique (RAO) projection and grafts to the right coronary artery (RCA) in a LAO projection.

Management of Saphenous Vein Graft Stenosis

Redo Coronary Artery Bypass Graft Versus Percutaneous Coronary Intervention

Repeat CABG carries a two- to four-fold higher risk of periprocedural death and myocardial infarctions (MI) compared to first-time CABG.[4] The presence of a patent left internal mammary artery (LIMA) to LAD makes redo CABG less beneficial compared to the initial CABG. On the other hand, PCI of native vessels has lower risk of periprocedural death and MI when compared to PCI of SVGs, and thus should be the initial strategy whenever feasible.[5]

Site of Lesions in the Grafts

- *Aorto-ostial lesions*: Percutaneous coronary intervention of aorto-ostial lesions has a restenosis rate of 42% compared to 17% with nonostial lesions. Final luminal diameter is the major determinant of restenosis following aorto-ostial PCI.

- *Lesions in the body of the graft*: Lesions in the body of the graft can be treated with stents with a higher success rate and a less than 5% complication rate.

- *Distal anastomotic lesions*: Due to mismatch between the graft and native vessel, stenting of the distal anastomotic lesion is difficult. Balloon angioplasty alone is very safe and effective, and probably the treatment of choice for these lesions.

Approach to Percutaneous Coronary Intervention of Saphenous Vein Graft Lesions

Figure 7c.1 shows the typical PCI of an SVG lesion.

Pharmacology (Antiplatelet and Antithrombotic Therapies) during SVG PCI

Heparin or bivalirudin is the antithrombotic agent of choice, with less bleeding associated with the latter's use. Studies have demonstrated that glycoprotein IIb/IIIa inhibitors may not be beneficial for PCI of SVG lesions.[5] A clopidogrel loading dose of 600 mg should be used at least 2 hours prior to an elective SVG intervention, if feasible, for better antiplatelet effects. Aspirin and clopidogrel maintenance therapy should then be continued.

Choice of Guide Catheters

Vein grafts with horizontal take-off, as is the case in most, can be engaged by a JR4 guide catheter. Right coronary grafts with inferior take-off are usually better engaged with a multipurpose guide catheter. Shape and tortuosity of the aorta are very important criteria when selecting a guide catheter. Although most of the left coronary grafts can be engaged with a JR4 catheter, in dilated and tortuous aorta, the Amplatz left (AL) or Amplatz right (AR) guides need to be used for left and right coronary engagement, respectively. Occasionally, a very superior take-off of a vein graft requires a specially designed bypass

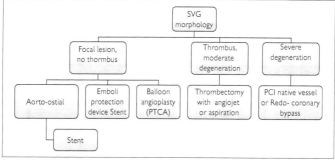

Figure 7c.1 Approach to the percutaneous coronary intervention of saphenous vein graft lesions based on the site and morphology. Adapted and reprinted from Freed M, Safian RD. *Manual of interventional cardiology*, 3rd ed. (Figure 17.5). Sudbury, MA: Jones and Barlett Publishers, 2001, with permission of the publisher (Jones and Barlett Publishers).

graft catheter (left or right coronary bypass graft catheters). When the lesion is ostial, and pressure dampening is noted during diagnostic angiogram, a guide catheter with side holes may be used to avoid impaired perfusion following catheter engagement.

Guidewire and Emboli Protection Devices

The advent of PercuSurge[6] and Filter Wire[7] emboli protection devices (EPDs; see Tables 7c.1 and 7c.2) heralded a new era in the PCI of SVG lesions. Use of these devices causes a significant reduction in major adverse cardiac events (42% relative risk reduction in major adverse events with PercuSurge device compared to conventional stenting). However, aorto-ostial lesions, lesions within 2.5 cm of distal anastomosis, vessel diameters of less than 3.5 mm and more than 5.5 mm, and less than 2 cm of straight vessel distal to lesion are exclusions for the use of some of these devices. Absence of adequate landing zone, smaller distal vessels, tight stenosis, and tortuous anatomy may make the delivery or use of embolic filter devices difficult. In these situations, proximal occlusion using Proxis EPDs may be useful, as they do not have these limitations and the thrombus can be aspirated even before the deployment of balloons or stents, thus minimizing the no-reflow phenomenon.[8]

Choice of Stents

Choice of stents in the treatment of SVG is controversial. Use of sirolimus-eluting stents reduces angiographic and clinical restenosis at 6 months compared to bare metal stents (BMSs).[9] However, when studied over longer periods, BMSs may tend to confer lower long-term mortality over drug-eluting stents (DESs).[10] The recently published PELOPS (Paclitaxel-Eluting Stent Long-term Outcomes in Percutaneous Saphenous Vein Graft Interventions) study concluded that implantation of PESs to

Table 7c.1 Pros and cons of different types of emboli protection devices

Device type	Pros	Cons
Filter emboli protection device (EPD)	Preserve antegrade flow throughout the procedure	May not capture debris smaller than pore size
	Optimal visualization of the lesion	Not as steerable as coronary wires
		May cause spasm or dissection
		Lesion crossing not protected
	Lesion crossing with guidewire of choice possible (with wire independent systems)	Filter may cause flow obstruction (slow flow, no flow)
		Due to stiffness of the device, may not be placed in the presence of excessive tortuosity
	Can be deployed and captured rapidly	Apposition in tortuous vessel may not be optimal
	Easy to use	
		Requires a vessel segment distal to the lesion suitable for placement (landing zone)
Proximal balloon occlusion ± flow reversal	All the steps of the procedures are protected	Transient flow obstruction may be poorly tolerated
	Crossing of the lesion with guidewire of choice	Poor visualization of the lesion
		Handling more demanding
	Protection also possible in presence of excessive tortuosity	Larger sheath size required
		Occlusive balloons may cause dissection or spasm
	Protection independent of particle size	Time-consuming set-up
Distal balloon occlusion	Protection independent of particle size	Transient flow obstruction may be poorly tolerated
	Lower profile and less stiff than filter EPD	Poor visualization of the lesion
		Crossing of the lesion not protected
	More easily delivered in tortuous anatomy	Use more cumbersome
		Potential for balloon induced injury
		Less steerable than coronary guidewire

Adapted from Roffi M, Abou-Chebl A, Mukherjee D, eds. *Principles of carotid artery stenting.* Bremen, Germany: Uni-Med, 2008:44-49, with permission of the publisher.

Table 7c.2 Predictors of 30–day outcomes during saphenous vein graft (SVG) intervention in emboli protection device trials

	Odds Ratio	95% Confidence Interval	p
Age (per 10 year)	1.21	1.07–1.37	0.01
Current smoker	1.50	1.08–2.08	0.01
Glycoprotein IIb/IIIa inhibitor use	1.30	1.03–1.64	0.03
Thrombus	1.62	1.24–2.11	0.0004
SVG degeneration Score (per category higher)	1.54	1.37–1.74	<0.0001
Plaque volume (per 100 mm³)	1.30	1.20–1.41	<0.0001

Reprinted from Coolong A. Saphenous vein graft stenting and major adverse cardiac events. A predictive model derived from a pooled analysis of 3958 patients. *Circulation.* 2008;117:790–797, adapted with permission of the publisher (Wolters Kluwer Health).

treat degenerative aortocoronary SVG lesions is safe and associated with low late loss, angiographic restenosis, and major adverse cardiac event (MACE) at 1-year follow-up.[11] The STENT (Strategic Transcatheter Evaluation of New Therapies) study suggested that the use of DESs compared with BMSs in SVG intervention is effective in reducing TVR in the short term, but most of this benefit seems to have been lost by 2 years. Furthermore, the short-term benefit seems to be most pronounced in SVGs with small reference lumen diameter (<3.5 mm), and there seems to be little or no benefit in SVGs with large reference lumen diameter.[12] Bare metal stents would be preferred in SVGs of greater than 3.5 mm in diameter, whereas DESs may have restenosis advantage in vessels that are smaller than 3.5 mm. Various stents are shown in Figures 7c.2–7c.4.

Complications of Percutaneous Coronary Intervention in Saphenous Vein Grafts

- *No reflow*: Distal embolization and no reflow occur at 5%–15% following SVG PCI. No reflow is more frequent in older (>3 years old) and degenerated vein grafts. Intracoronary nitroprusside, intracoronary adenosine, or calcium channel blockers (nicardipine or verapamil) help prevent/treat the no-reflow phenomenon. Distal EPDs are also effective in reducing no-reflow phenomenon.

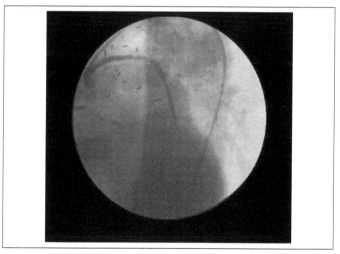

Figure 7c.2 A thrombotic lesion in the body of a vein graft prior to intervention. Reprinted from Coolong A. Saphenous vein graft stenting and major adverse cardiac events. A predictive model derived from a pooled analysis of 3,958 patients. *Circulation.* 2008;117:790-797, with permission of the publisher (Wolters Kluwer Health).

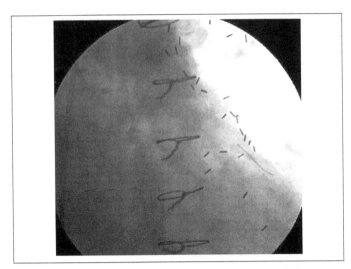

Figure 7c.3 Deployment of an emboli protection device in a vein graft during intervention.

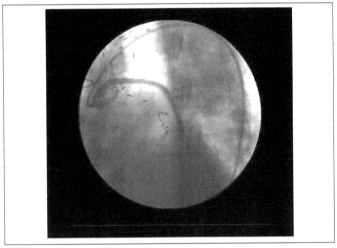

Figure 7c.4 Final angiogram of a vein graft lesion after placement of a bare metal stent.

- *Abrupt closure*: Abrupt closure occurs in 1%–2% of PCI involving SVGs. It is usually caused by dissection and can often be treated by stenting of the dissection.

- *Perforation*: Although rare, perforation can occur during the use of now-defunct atherectomy devices. Emergency surgery or Jo-Med stents can be used to seal the perforation.

- *Restenosis*: Ostial and proximal lesions, diffuse lesions, small vessels, chronic total occlusion, and older grafts (>3 years) are predictors of restenosis, which occurs in 23%–73% at 6 months.

Special Considerations

Chronic total occlusions (CTOs) of an SVG are universally associated with large thrombus burden, and thus PCI of an SVG CTO is met with lowest procedural success and the highest risk of periprocedural MI and death. Thus, PCI of native vessels must always be tried before attempting to intervene on a CTO of an SVG.

Conclusion

Percutaneous coronary intervention of SVGs is a high-risk intervention. No reflow occurs more frequently with SVG intervention compared to native-vessel PCI. Lesion preparation with the use of EPDs and liberal use of preprocedural intracoronary vasodilators such as adenosine, calcium channel blockers (nicardipine), or nitroprusside may help minimize this phenomenon. Choice of stent must be individualized, based on the lesion type and lesion diameter.

Practical Pearls

- Balloon angioplasty followed by stenting is ideal for SVG lesions at the aorto-ostial site and at the body of the graft.

- Balloon angioplasty alone may suffice for distal anastomotic lesions.

- Direct stenting may help minimize the risks of distal embolization and no reflow.

- Whenever feasible, attempts to intervene on the native vessel are more prudent than PCI of degenerated vein grafts.

- Embolic protection devices are very effective in reducing distal embolization with SVG PCI and should be used.

- Pretreatment of the vein graft with intracoronary calcium channel blocker use (e.g., nicardipine) may reduce the incidence of no-reflow.

References

1. Morwani JG, Topol EJ. Aortocoronary saphenous vein graft disease pathogenesis, predispositions, and prevention. *Circulation.* 1998;97:916-931.

2. Reul GJ, Cooley DA, Ott DA, et al. Reoperation for recurrent coronary artery disease. *Arch Surg.* 1979;114:1269-1275.

3. Douglas JS, Weintraub WS, Liberman HA, et al. Update of saphenous graft (SVG) angioplasty: restenosis and long term outcome. *Circulation.* 1991;84:II-249.

4. Foster E, Fisher L, Kaiser G, et al. Comparison of operative mortality and morbidity for initial and repeat coronary artery bypass grafting. The CASS registry experience. *Ann Thorac Surg.* 1984;35:563-570.

5. Roffi M, Mikherjee D, Chew DP, et al. Lack of benefit from intravenous platelet glycoprotein IIb/IIIa receptor inhibition as adjunctive treatment for percutaneous interventions of aortocoronary bypass grafts: a pooled analysis of five randomized clinical trials. *Circulation.* 2002;106:3063-3067.

6. Baim DS, Wahr D, George B, et al., on behalf of the Saphenous Vein Graft Angioplasty Free of Emboli Randomized (SAFER) Trial investigators. Randomized trial of a distal embolic protection device during percutaneous intervention of saphenous vein aorto-coronary grafts. *Circulation.* 2002;105:1285-1290.

7. Stone GW, Rogers C, Ramee S, et al. Distal filter protection during saphenous vein graft stenting: technical and clinical correlates of efficacy. *J Am Coll Cardiol.* 2002;40:1882-1888.

8. Mauri L, Cox D, Hermiller J, et al. The PROXIMAL trial: Proximal protection during saphenous vein graft intervention using the Proxis Embolic Protection System: a randomized, prospective, multicenter clinical trial. *J Am Coll Cardiol.* 2007;50:1442-1449.

9. Vermeersch P, Agostoni P, Verheye S, et al. Randomized, controlled blind comparison of sirolimus-eluting stent versus bare-metal stent implantation in diseased saphenous vein grafts: six-month angiographic, intravascular ultrasound, and clinical follow-up of the RRISC Trial. *J Am Coll Cardiol.* 2006;48:2423-2431.

10. Vermeersch P, Agostoni P, Verheye S, et al. Increased late mortality after sirolimus-eluting stents versus bare-metal stents in diseased saphenous vein grafts: results from the randomized DELAYED RRISC trial. *J Am Coll Cardiol.* 2007;50:261-267.

11. Jim MH, Ho HH, Ko RL, Yiu KH, Siu CW, Lau CP, Chow WH. Paclitaxel-eluting stent long-term outcomes in percutaneous saphenous vein graft interventions (PELOPS) study. *Am J Cardiol.* 2009;103:199-202.

12. Brodie BR, Wilson H, Stuckey T et al for the STENT Group Outcomes With Drug-Eluting Versus Bare-Metal Stents in Saphenous Vein Graft Intervention: results from the STENT (Strategic Transcatheter Evaluation of New Therapies) group *J Am Coll Cardiol Intv* 2009;2:1035-1046 .

Chapter 7d

Chronic Total Occlusion

Khaled M. Ziada

Percutaneous coronary intervention (PCI) of chronic total occlusion (CTO) is one of the most challenging subsets of angioplasty encountered by interventional cardiologists today. Depending on the referral patterns, CTO PCI can represent 5%–20% of the PCI volume in busy catheterization laboratories. Nonetheless, CTO remains a major indication for referral to surgical revascularization in the United States.[1]

Performance of such procedures should be carefully considered by the interventional operator and the patient (Table 7d.1).[2] It is generally preferred to schedule CTO PCI rather than proceed with ad hoc interventions (as is more common with non-CTO PCI)[3]. This allows better consideration of optimization of medical therapy, expected benefits, and risk of complications.

This chapter focuses on the step-by-step technical approach to the performance of CTO PCI.

Arterial Access

Traditionally, femoral access is preferred to radial or brachial access in CTO PCI, primarily for better support and because of the need for dual access in some cases (Table 7d.2). Operators highly experienced in the radial approach find no significant disadvantage in that approach in properly selected cases.[4]

Anticoagulation

Because of the potential risk of perforation with the use of stiff CTO wires, anticoagulants should be readily reversible. Intravenous unfractionated heparin remains the preferred anticoagulant for CTO PCI. Activated clotting time (ACT) should be frequently checked and maintained in a therapeutic range (>250 sec) due to the length of the procedure and the possibility of multiple wire or balloon catheter use in the guiding catheter lumen. It is reasonable to preload patients with clopidogrel or other thienopyridines prior to the procedure for effective antiplatelet effects. The use of intravenous glycoprotein IIb/IIIa inhibitors is not preferred, at least until the wire safely crosses into the distal true lumen.

Table 7d.1 Considerations in deciding to proceed with chronic total occlusion (CTO) percutaneous coronary intervention (PCI)

- Clear indication and potential for benefit[2]
- Is the procedure expected to relieve significant angina or angina-equivalent symptoms despite optimal medical therapy?

OR

- Is there evidence of significant areas of ischemia on an imaging functional study?

OR

- Is there potential for improvement in regional myocardial function (i.e., evidence of viability and hibernation)?

OR

- Is there a potential survival benefit?[3]
- Clear and informed consent.
- Although recently improved, CTO PCI success rates are significantly lower than standard PCI.
- While the risk of major adverse events is not significantly higher with CTO PCI, the potential for complications does exist and should be balanced against the expected benefit.
- There may be a need for more than one procedure to achieve success.
- There is a risk of excessive radiation exposure and use of large volumes of contrast.
- The decision to proceed with CTO PCI and the likelihood of success are influenced by the technical experience of the interventional operator.[2]

Table 7d.2 Considerations of arterial access in chronic total occlusion (CTO) percutaneous coronary intervention (PCI)

- 7 or 8 Fr guiding catheters are almost always needed for better backup support.
- Potential need for use of anchoring balloon system to stabilize the guiding catheter
- Potential need for use of IVUS imaging (across a branching point) to guide CTO wire
- Dual arterial access (via both femoral arteries) may be needed to visualize retrograde collateral filling from the contralateral artery, facilitating direction of CTO wire in case of retrograde approaches requiring guiding catheters in both coronary arteries.
- Long (45 or 65 cm) rigid sheaths can enhance backup support.

IVUS, intravenous ultrasound.

Guide Catheter Selection

Chronic total occlusion PCI requires significant backup support to allow advancing balloons and subsequently stents through the occluded segment[5]. Since passing the wire is usually the most difficult step, the selected catheter must be used from the beginning of the procedure. Various catheter shapes can be selected, with backup support being the critical determinant (Table 7d.3). In almost all cases of CTO PCI, a 7 or 8 Fr guiding catheter is preferred. This improves backup support and allows the use of advanced techniques such as

Table 7d.3 Guiding catheter shapes for chronic total occlusion (CTO) percutaneous coronary intervention (PCI)

- Right Coronary Artery CTO
  - Best backup support: AL1 or AL0.75
  - Moderate support: AR shapes
  - Least support: JR shapes
- Left Coronary Artery CTO
  - Best backup support: AL2, AL1, or Extra-backup shapes
  - Moderate or weak support: JL shapes
- When using guiding catheters with moderate or weak backup support, an anchoring balloon system can enhance the stability of the guide and the ability to advance through the CTO (see Fig. 7d.1). This is helpful in cases of proximal or ostial disease, in which more aggressive guide catheter shapes cannot be used.

balloon anchoring and intravascular ultrasound (IVUS)-guided wiring of the CTO segment. In retrograde techniques, short catheters (≤90 cm) are needed to increase the working shaft length of microcatheters or balloon catheters.

Wires and Wiring Techniques

Several new techniques of CTO PCI have recently been developed, primarily by experienced Japanese operators. In addition, wire technology has markedly advanced, leading to a wide variety of dedicated CTO wires (Table 7d.4). This allows interventionists to tackle cases that were not previously considered feasible and hence improves the success rates appreciably.

Antegrade Techniques

Single-wire Technique

The mainstay of CTO PCI remains similar to standard PCI (i.e., antegrade advancement of a single wire from the proximal true lumen to the distal true lumen). Important differences in angiography and technique are outlined in Table 7d.5. An over-the-wire balloon or a microcatheter is advanced over any soft or moderately stiff wire to the site of the CTO. At that point, the wire is replaced by the special CTO wire of choice. This maneuver protects the proximal vessel from the stiff CTO wire and allows the operator to shape the tip of the CTO wire more appropriately (much smaller bend, closer to the tip). A graduated wire approach is usually followed, starting with a softer wire and progressing to stiffer ones as needed. Having the balloon or the microcatheter close to the tip of the wire increases its stiffness significantly. Experienced operators may prefer going directly to stiffer specialty wires to reduce the risk of creating a false channel with softer wires.

Table 7d.4 Commonly used chronic total occlusion wires currently available in the United States[2]

Manufacturer	Wire	Tip Stiffness (g)	Shaft and Tip Diameter (inches)
Asahi/Abbott	Whisper	1	0.014
	Medium	3	0.014
	Fielder	1	0.014
	Fielder FC	1	0.014–0.009
	Fielder XT	1	0.014
	Miracle Bros.	3, 4.5, 6, 12	0.014
	Confianza	9, 12	0.014–0.009
	Confianza Pro	9, 12	0.014–0.009
	Pilot 50, 150, 200	1.6, 3, 4.5	0.014
Medtronic	Persuader	3, 6	0.014
	Persuader 9	9	0.014–0.009
Boston Scientific	Choice PT	2	0.014
	PT Graphix	3–4	0.014
Cordis	Shinobi	2	0.014
	Shinobi Plus	4	0.014

Table 7d.5 Angiographic and technical considerations unique to chronic total occlusion (CTO) percutaneous coronary intervention (PCI)

- Estimation of a reasonable trajectory from the proximal stump to the distal true lumen
- High-quality angiograms obtained in different views for definition of branches, branching points, calcification, and bridging collateral vessels
- High-quality angiograms of the contralateral vessel to define retrograde collaterals and extent of retrograde filling. Dual simultaneous right and left coronary injections can be of great help.
- Some of these goals can be achieved by coronary computed tomography (CT) angiography performed for planning a few days prior to the scheduled PCI.[5]
- An over-the-wire system (microcatheter or balloon) should be used to allow wire exchanges through the lumen without losing position within the artery.
- Provide further stiffness to the wire by advancing the shaft of the catheter closer to the wire tip.
- Confirm position in true lumen after crossing.
- CTO wire manipulation is distinctly different from usual PCI.
- The tip is very short and the angle is also very narrow (i.e., the wire tip is very close to being straight).
- To penetrate CTO, the motion is mostly piercing and burrowing with some aiming and direction (opposite of non-CTO PCI technique).

As the wire is advanced into the CTO segment, several possibilities exist and the clinical experience of the operator cannot be overemphasized. Figure 7d.1 provides a general outline of the possibilities and the tools that can be used at each decision point.

If the stiff CTO wire is successfully advanced into the true lumen, it should be replaced by a moderate support wire to avoid potential injury to the distal vessel during percutaneous transluminal coronary angioplasty (PTCA) and stenting (Fig. 7d.2). Frequently, distal segments are diffusely diseased, and multiple and/or long stents are required. Commonly, distal vessels appear small due to underfilling and impaired endothelial function. This should be considered when deciding on the size of stents to be used.

After the wire is advanced beyond the CTO segment, several clues can be used to recognize the location of the wire, whether in the true lumen or subintimal track (Table 7d.6 and Fig. 7d.3). This is a critical step prior to advancing the balloon or the microcatheter into the distal vessel and proceeding with PTCA and stenting.

113

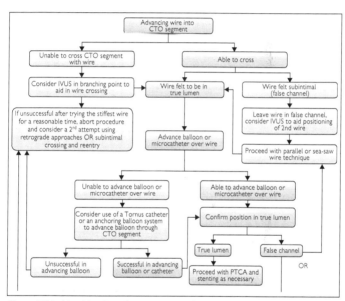

Figure 7d.1 Algorithm for utilizing various tools and approaches during chronic total occlusion percutaneous coronary intervention.

Table 7d.6 Clues to identifying true lumen (vs. subintimal course) after wire crosses chronic total occlusion

- Experienced operators are usually able to determine the location by tactile feel and freedom of tip motion.
- The ability to advance wire in more than one anatomically expected distal branches.
- Inject contrast in the contralateral vessel to fill retrograde collaterals and locate the tip of the wire in relation to the retrogradely filled distal vessel in multiple projections.
- Advance the balloon or microcatheter and inject contrast through the wire lumen to visualize the distal lumen (see Fig. 7d.3).

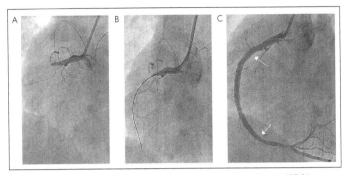

Figure 7d.2 Example of right coronary artery chronic total occlusion (CTO) percutaneous coronary intervention using the single-wire technique. (A) The proximal stump appears favorable for directing the wire tip, and the bridging collaterals faintly fill the mid vessel, helping direct the wire. Retrograde filling from left to right collaterals reached the distal segment of the artery (not shown). (B) A Miracle Bros™ wire (weight tip 3 g) was advanced through the CTO segment without significant difficulty. Note the very subtle bend on the tip of the wire. (C) After the wire is advanced to the distal vessel and percutaneous transluminal coronary angioplasty (PTCA) is performed, there is significant disease involving the entire mid vessel, which was eventually stented (*arrows*) with a satisfactory angiographic result.

The ability to advance a balloon into the CTO segment for an initial PTCA can be challenging in some cases due to the marked calcification, tortuosity, and/or inadequate guide catheter support. Low-profile microcatheters and small balloons with no distal markers have a better chance of crossing than do regular double-marker PTCA balloons. If unsuccessful, the Tornus™ catheter can be used to burrow through the lesion by carefully advancing and rotating it in a counterclockwise direction (Fig. 7d.4).

Double-wire Technique

The double-wire approach is the most common secondary technique used when the first attempt of crossing the CTO with the wire ends in a subintimal false channel (see Fig. 7d.1). In such cases, the wire should be left in place for two purposes: to plug the entrance to the false channel, and, with angiography in multiple projections, to guide the entrance of a second wire (Figs. 7d.5 and 7d.6). Generally, CTO wires pass into false channels because of failure to follow a natural angulation (i.e., they tend to follow the outer curvature when they are supposed to follow the inner curvature of a vessel). Therefore, the second wire almost always needs to be on the inside of the first one (i.e., the ventricular side in the case of a right coronary artery [RCA] CTO and septal side the in case of a left anterior descending [LAD] artery).

If the second wire again passes into a false channel, it can be left in place and the first one pulled back and used for another attempt, hence the name *see-saw technique*. Other operators prefer to leave both wires in place and try to cross with a third wire.

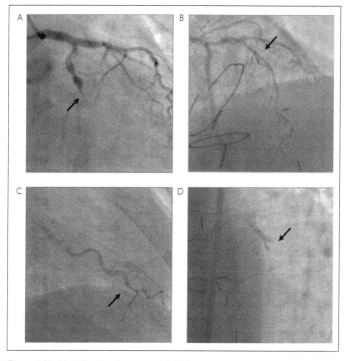

Figure 7d.3 Identification of true versus false lumen using the wire lumen of the balloon catheter. After crossing with the wire, a small balloon or microcatheter is advanced distal to the chronic total occlusion (CTO) segment. The wire is then removed and contrast is injected into the wire lumen. Before injecting, it is important to ensure the lumen is cleared of air by giving it time to "bleed back," aspirating gently using a small syringe and filling the catheter hub with saline as a small contrast syringe is connected. Immediately after the contrast injection, the lumen must be cleared by a saline injection to avoid crystallization of contrast molecules, which can impair advancing the wire back in the distal lumen. (A and B) An example of CTO of the obtuse marginal (OM) branch of left circumflex (LCX). The balloon is in the true lumen, as evidenced by brisk flow and washout of contrast, in addition to visualization of small branches distally (B, *arrow*). (C and D) In comparison, after crossing this complex CTO of the mid left anterior descending (LAD) artery (*arrow*, beyond origin of second septal and a diagonal branch), the balloon is in a subintimal track, which is irregular, has no branches, and "stains" with contrast.

Retrograde Technique

This technique utilizes the collaterals from the contralateral artery to access the distal cap of the CTO plaque, when antegrade penetration of the CTO was attempted without success or if it is considered unlikely to succeed (such as with an ostial CTO, very long CTO, or marked proximal tortuosity).[2,6] The most commonly used collaterals include septal perforators (from LAD to RCA

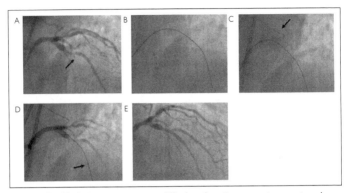

Figure 7d.4 Techniques to overcome difficulty advancing a percutaneous transluminal coronary angioplasty (PTCA) catheter across chronic total occlusion (CTO) segment. (A) Although the operator selected an 8 Fr AL2 guiding catheter and the wire crossed the mid left anterior descending (LAD) CTO (*arrow*), a balloon could not be advanced. Two maneuvers were used simultaneously, although each can be tried separately. (B) A Tornus™ catheter is used to burrow forward into the occluded segment, but with no success due to inadequate support. (C) An anchoring balloon is then advanced in a small left circumflex (LCX) branch (*arrow*) and inflated to stabilize the guiding catheter. (D) The subsequent forward pressure with the Tornus catheter is successful and the lesion is crossed. (E) The final result after stenting of the LAD and PTCA of the diagonal branch.

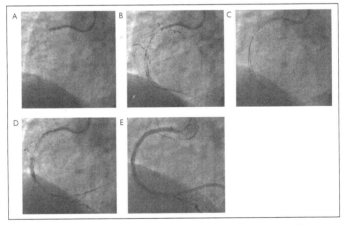

Figure 7d.5 Double-wire technique. (A) In this example of chronic total occlusion (CTO) right coronary artery (RCA), an 8 Fr AL1 guide is used. (B) The first wire enters into a false channel. (C) The wire is left in place, and a second wire (of similar or higher stiffness, but shaped slightly differently) is advanced on the inner curvature of the artery (*arrow*). (D) The wire enters the true lumen and, after percutaneous transluminal coronary angioplasty (PTCA), severe diffuse disease is appreciated. (E) Further PTCA and stenting leads to the final result.

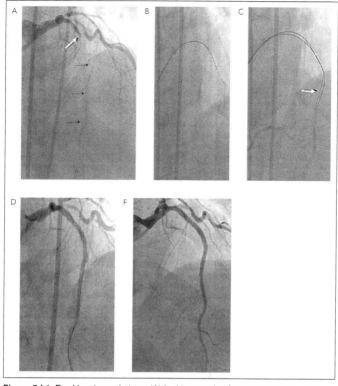

Figure 7d.6 Double-wire technique. (A) In this example of percutaneous coronary intervention of chronic total occlusion (CTO) in the mid left anterior descending (LAD) artery, dual right and left coronary injections are used to define the length of the occluded segment (*white arrow*: antegrade stump; *black arrow*: R>L collateral filling) and provide guidance for advancing the antegrade wire. (B) The first wire enters a false channel, which can be determined by the retrograde injection from the right coronary artery (RCA) catheter. (C) The second wire is directed "inward" (i.e., on the septal side of the first) and enters the true lumen. (D) The final result after percutaneous transluminal coronary angioplasty and stenting, and (E) a follow-up angiogram after 3 months demonstrates continued patency.

and vice versa), epicardial and atrial collaterals. Defining the collateral anatomy frequently requires subselective injections using PTCA catheters or microcatheters advanced into the collateral vessel. Defining the actual size, degree of tortuosity, and continuity of the collateral with the recipient vessel are all critical steps in planning the procedure. These vessels are thin walled and more prone to dissection and rupture, thus wiring should be done meticulously and with patience (Fig. 7d.7a–h).

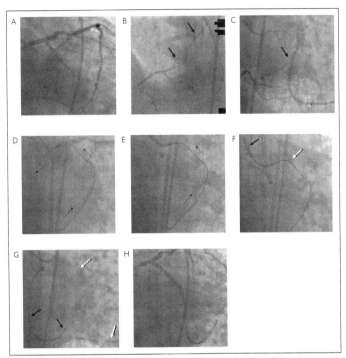

Figure 7d.7 Example of retrograde chronic total occlusion (CTO) percutaneous coronary intervention (PCI) of left circumflex (LCX). (A) In addition to CTO in the proximal segment, there is severe calcification at the ostium, and the left main artery is diseased. An attempt at antegrade PCI has previously failed. (B) The epicardial collateral from the PL branch of right coronary artery along the anteroventral (AV) groove is relatively straight and of good size (*arrows*). (C) The angle between the collateral and the recipient LCX is favorable that is, it directs the wire towards the CTO segment (*arrow*). In retrograde CTO PCI, guiding catheters need to be short (90 cm or slightly less if the catheter is cut manually) to have a longer working balloon shaft length. Dual coronary injections are then performed to define the collaterals and the recipient segment distal to the CTO (A–C). A soft wire is advanced into the collateral through a balloon catheter or a microcatheter. Septal perforators tend to spasm over the wire and frequently require very gentle balloon inflations (1.25 or 1.5 mm balloon at 1–2 atm). A septal dilator catheter is now available and may obviate the need for this step. (D) The balloon or microcatheter is then advanced into the distal recipient vessel, and the soft wire is removed for a stiffer wire. (E) The CTO cap is penetrated from distal to proximal, and the retrograde wire is advanced into the antegrade guiding catheter. (F) Percutaneous transluminal coronary angioplasty (PTCA) of the CTO is then performed by advancing the retrograde balloon (white arrow). (F) This can be facilitated by stabilizing the retrograde wire in the antegrade guiding catheter using a balloon inflated in the body of the catheter (*black arrow*). (G) After PTCA, a channel is created, an antegrade wire is advanced (*white arrow*), while the retrograde wire (*black arrow*) is removed. (H) The procedure is completed (further PTCA and stenting) via the antegrade guiding catheter.

Subintimal Tracking and Reentry Techniques

This group of techniques can be performed antegrade or retrograde. They are generally reserved for cases that are not amenable to the techniques described earlier. In brief, a wire is used to intentionally create a dissection plane that extends into the arterial wall from the proximal stump to the distal vessel, spanning the length of the CTO segment. Another wire, generally a very stiff specialty CTO wire, is then advanced into the dissection plane and used to reenter the true lumen beyond the CTO. This can be facilitated by IVUS imaging from the dissection plane, which can better identify the direction of reentry; dedicated IVUS imaging and reentry systems have been developed for coronary as well as peripheral occlusions. New devices, such as the CrossBoss™, have recently been approved to facilitate that approach. After reentry, PTCA and stenting can be performed in the usual manner, although the majority of the stented segments will be subintimal.

Success Rates and Complications

Chronic total occlusion PCI success rates have improved from the traditional 70% range to more than 85% in recent reports incorporating aggressive and contemporary techniques.[7,8] In a recent report, the procedural success rate of the retrograde approach was 65%, but it could be increased to 85% with adjunctive use of antegrade and subintimal tracking techniques.[6] Despite improvement, there is no evidence of an increase in attempts at CTO PCI.[2] Several angiographic characteristics can predict lower likelihood of success (Table 7d.7).

The incidence of major adverse events has significantly dropped over the last few decades. Death, emergent surgery, and Q-wave myocardial infarction (MI) are rare (<1.0%). Non-Q wave MIs occur 1%–3% more when the CTO PCI is successful.[9] Most concerning is coronary perforation, which is significantly more frequent with CTO PCI than with standard PCI. In the Total Occlusion Angioplasty Study-Società Italiana di Cardiologia Invasiva (TOAST-GISE) study, successful PCI was achieved in a high percentage of CTOs with a low incidence of immediate complications. Furthermore, at 1-year follow-up, patients with

---

Table 7d.7 Angiographic predictors of failure of chronic total occlusion (CTO) percutaneous coronary intervention

- Antegrade Techniques[9,10]
  - CTO >15 mm, severe calcification, severe proximal tortuosity, side branch at site of CTO, bridging collaterals
- Retrograde Techniques[6]
- Failure to cross the collateral vessel (marked tortuosity, failure to visualize connection between collateral and recipient vessel, and/or unfavorable angle between collateral and recipient vessel)

successful PCI of a CTO had a significantly better clinical outcome than those whose PCI was unsuccessful[10]. The absolute incidence of complications remains low in other studies (0.9%) and with no evidence of increased mortality.[11] With complex techniques incorporating multiple stiff wires and instrumentation of collateral vessels, the incidence of perforation is much higher (up to 11%).[8] These are mostly type 1 perforations, caused by wire exit distal to the CTO segment, thus not resulting in clinical consequences in the majority of cases. Attention must be paid to delayed tamponade, diagnosed hours after the procedure, which is a typical presentation for wire perforations.

Due to the complexity and length of CTO PCI procedures, patients and operators are exposed to higher doses of radiation.[12] Efforts should be made to reduce both patient (collimation, reduced frame rate, and changing intensifier position) and operator exposure (accessory lead shields, right anterior oblique [RAO] projections, reduced frame rate).[2] Patients should be informed about such risk prior to the procedure, and failure of PCI should be accepted if fluoroscopy time exceeds 60 minutes without significant progress.

For similar reasons, contrast load is higher in CTO PCI. Operators should be restrained when using contrast during wiring and in cases in which dual injections are needed. Ideally, CTO PCI is scheduled so that patients are well hydrated and the procedure planning can be based on prior angiograms.

Conclusion

Chronic total occlusion PCI remains a significant challenge in contemporary interventional cardiology. Success rates have improved significantly, but vast experience is needed to achieve these improved outcomes. Nonetheless, the potential for complications exists, particularly with more aggressive and complex techniques. Prior to attempting these procedures, operators and patients need to have a comprehensive discussion about risks versus benefits.

Practical Pearls

- Although recently improved, CTO PCI success rates are significantly lower than those for standard PCI.
- 7 or 8 Fr guiding catheters are almost always needed for better backup support.
- Unfractionated heparin remains the preferred anticoagulant for CTO PCI.
- An over-the-wire system (microcatheter or balloon) should be used to allow wire exchanges through the lumen without losing position within the artery.
- To penetrate the CTO, the guidewire motion is mostly piercing and burrowing, with some aiming and direction (opposite of non-CTO PCI technique).
- Attention must be paid to delayed tamponade, diagnosed hours after the procedure, which is a typical presentation for wire perforations.

References

1. Christofferson RD, Lehmann KG, Martin GV, Every N, Caldwell JH, Kapadia SR. Effect of chronic total coronary occlusion on treatment strategy. *Am J Cardiol.* 2005;95:1088-1091.

2. Grantham JA, Marso SP, Spertus J, House J, Holmes DR, Jr., Rutherford BD. Chronic total occlusion angioplasty in the United States. *JACC Cardiovasc Interv.* 2009;2:479-486.

3. Safley DM, House JA, Marso SP, Grantham JA, Rutherford BD. Improvement in survival following successful percutaneous coronary intervention of coronary chronic total occlusions: variability by target vessel. *JACC Cardiovasc Interv.* 2008;1:295-302.

4. Rathore S, Hakeem A, Pauriah M, Roberts E, Beaumont A, Morris JL. A comparison of the transradial and the transfemoral approach in chronic total occlusion percutaneous coronary intervention. *Catheter Cardiovasc Interv.* 2009;73:883-887.

5. Hoe J. CT coronary angiography of chronic total occlusions of the coronary arteries: How to recognize and evaluate and usefulness for planning percutaneous coronary interventions. *Int J Cardiovasc Imaging.* 2009;25(Suppl 1):43-54.

6. Rathore S, Katoh O, Matsuo H, et al. Retrograde percutaneous recanalization of chronic total occlusion of the coronary arteries: procedural outcomes and predictors of success in contemporary practice. *Circ Cardiovasc Intervent.* 2009;2:124-132.

7. Prasad A, Rihal CS, Lennon RJ, Wiste HJ, Singh M, Holmes DR, Jr. Trends in outcomes after percutaneous coronary intervention for chronic total occlusions: a 25-year experience from the Mayo Clinic. *J Am Coll Cardiol.* 2007;49:1611-1168.

8. Rathore S, Matsuo H, Terashima M, et al. Procedural and in-hospital outcomes after percutaneous coronary intervention for chronic total occlusions of coronary arteries 2002 to 2008: impact of novel guidewire techniques. *JACC Cardiovasc Interv.* 2009;2:489-497.

9. Suero JA, Marso SP, Jones PG, et al. Procedural outcomes and long-term survival among patients undergoing percutaneous coronary intervention of a chronic total occlusion in native coronary arteries: a 20-year experience. *J Am Coll Cardiol.* 2001;38:409-414.

10. Olivari Z, Rubartelli P, Piscione F, et al. Immediate results and one-year clinical outcome after percutaneous coronary interventions in chronic total occlusions: data from a multicenter, prospective, observational study (TOAST-GISE). *J Am Coll Cardiol.* 2003;41:1672-1678.

11. Javaid A, Buch AN, Satler LF, et al. Management and outcomes of coronary artery perforation during percutaneous coronary intervention. *Am J Cardiol.* 2006;98:911-914.

12. Suzuki S, Furui S, Kohtake H, et al. Radiation exposure to patient's skin during percutaneous coronary intervention for various lesions, including chronic total occlusion. *Circ J.* 2006;70:44-48.

Chapter 7e

Calcified Coronary Lesions

Sanjay Bhojraj and Adam Greenbaum

The management of calcified coronary arteries poses a unique set of challenges for the interventional cardiologist. Historically, percutaneous coronary intervention (PCI) of calcified lesions has been associated with lower success rates and worse outcomes.[1] Failure to deliver catheters, balloon rupture, vessel dissection, and failure to achieve a final percent diameter stenosis of less than 20% all occur more commonly during PCI of calcified lesions. Higher frequency of stent malapposition and asymmetry may account for higher acute and subacute stent thrombosis rates.[2] Even after successful stent placement, smaller luminal diameter and acute gain results in more frequent restenosis.[3] Various technologies and techniques may increase success and outcomes following PCI of calcified lesions.

Patient Management

Approach to the Patient

The first step in approaching the patient with coronary calcification is identification. A quick review of any recent computed tomography (CT) scan of the thorax can afford insight into the presence of coronary calcium. As CT coronary angiography gains more traction, patients may present with an in-depth analysis of the location and degree of calcification. Once identified, the next step is to ascertain whether the calcification will interfere with the delivery and performance of interventional equipment.

- *Intravascular ultrasound*: Conventional angiography is remarkably poor in visualizing coronary calcification, making it difficult to predict the complexity of treating these lesions.[4] The adoption of intravascular ultrasound (IVUS) has given the interventional cardiologist a more complete view of the calcified coronary plaque, allowing the perspective of both depth (intimal, medial, or adventitial) as well as the degree (arc) of coronary calcification (Fig. 7e.1).[5] Although all types of calcification will affect the delivery of equipment and acute gain, intimal and circumferential types may be particularly problematic

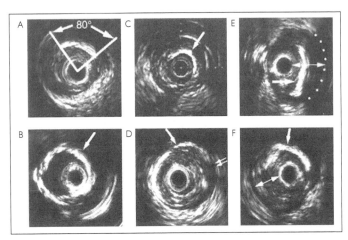

Figure 7e.1 Appearance of coronary calcium on intravascular ultrasound imaging. (A) Arc of target lesion calcium. (B) Circumferential, intimal calcium. (C) Arc of superficial calcium. (D) Circumferential, adventitial calcium. (E) Arc of adventitial calcium. (F) Arc of adventitial calcium perpendicular to the maximum plaque thickness. Reprinted from Mintz et al., *Circulation.* 1995;91:1959-1965, with permission of the publisher (American Heart Association, Inc./Elsevier).

and may prompt a change in strategy to "upfront" rotational atherectomy (RA) rather than reserving it for failure of the lesion to yield with high-pressure dilation. We recommend routinely starting with an IVUS analysis of calcification.

- *Guiding catheters*: Because of lower vessel compliance and increased rigidity, coronary calcium results in more difficult product delivery. In general, larger guiding catheters and "extra backup" shapes that offer greater support are preferred (Table 7e.1). Although up to a 1.75 mm RA burr for plaque "modification" can be delivered through some of the larger lumen (≥0.070-inch) 6 Fr guiding catheters, we recommend at least 7 Fr and preferably 8 Fr guiding catheters for more aggressive debulking with larger burr sizes, particularly when bare metal stent (BMS) use is planned, and/or for additional support.

- *Guidewires*: Use of stiffer guidewires may be required to successfully deliver equipment. In general, medium support wires are recommended. However, in cases of vessel tortuosity and/or angulated lesions, it may be difficult to cross a heavily calcified lesion with a supportive wire. In these cases, crossing a lesion with a light support or hydrophilic-coated wire and exchanging for the more supportive wire with an exchange catheter or an over-the-wire balloon system may be advantageous. Similarly, the less supportive 0.009-inch Rotafloppy™ wire (Boston Scientific, Natick, MA) may be difficult to primarily deliver and can also be exchanged for after successful delivery of

Table 7e.1 Guiding catheters useful during percutaneous intervention of calcified coronary lesions

Manufacturer	Left Coronary System	Right Coronary System
Abbott Vascular	GL JCL	GR
Boston Scientific	VODA Q-Curve CLS Kiesz	ART Kiesz
Cordis	XB XBLAD	XBRCA
Medtronic	EBU JCL	RBU
All Manufacturers	Amplatz Left	Amplatz Left

JCL, Judkins curved left; CLS, contralateral support.

a light support or hydrophilic 0.014-inch wire. If it still proves difficult to advance equipment past a calcified lesion, advancing a second guidewire (a "buddy wire") to assist has been established as a useful technique to deliver equipment. Another wire of potential benefit is the Wiggle™ Wire (Abbott Vascular, Abbott Park, IL), which can aid in delivery of products past eccentric intimal calcification via intentional bias away from the calcium. Rarely, medium-support wires in the setting of calcification combined with tortuosity may paradoxically hinder delivery of equipment. In these cases, reverting back to light support wires can occasionally lead to success not achievable with more supportive wires.

- *Dilation catheters*: In general, it will require noncompliant balloons and higher pressures to achieve adequate dilation of a calcified vessel for stent delivery and deployment. However, noncompliant balloons may not initially cross a calcified stenosis, and initial dilation with an undersized (0.75 balloon:artery ratio), more compliant balloon, even if the lesion fails to completely yield, may allow subsequent delivery of a noncompliant balloon. As very high-pressure predilation with a noncompliant balloon may result in major dissection contraindicating subsequent rotational atherectomy, we recommend a low threshold for converting to RA after failure of the lesion to yield with more moderate pressure dilation with a noncompliant balloon.

- *Stents*: Delivery of stents into heavily calcified lesions can be difficult and may result in procedural complications. In choosing a stent, the ability to cross a lesion is an important consideration and, in general, those stents with more compliant delivery systems are more deliverable. Yet stent apposition and symmetry are important in reducing acute and subacute complications, and a less compliant stent delivery system may be advantageous in the setting of vessel calcification. Therefore, stent choice should be deliberate and individualized. Given the smaller acute gain and maximal vessel diameter anticipated when treating calcified stenoses, drug-eluting stents (DESs) are generally preferred over BMSs.

Special Equipment

Prior to the widespread use of the DES, a major obstacle in treating calcified lesions was establishing a lumen large enough to avoid restenosis. This led to a proliferation of technologies aimed at increasing luminal diameter prior to stent insertion (Table 7e.2). With the advent of DES and reductions in late loss, the major remaining obstacle in treating calcified coronary lesions is more related to the delivery of the therapeutic equipment rather than maximizing luminal diameter.

• *Rotational atherectomy (RA)*: The Rotablator™ (Boston Scientific, Natick, MA) has established itself as invaluable in the delivery of interventional equipment through heavily calcified lesions. This device consists of a nickel-plated burr that is coated with 20–30 µm diamond chips attached to a flexible drive shaft covered by a Teflon sheath.[6] This burr rotates at 140,000–150,000 rpm and pulverizes coronary calcium into microparticles that are then taken up in the reticuloendothelial system.[7] Although acute procedural success is higher with RA, there has been a lack of definitive evidence demonstrating improvement in long-term outcomes.[8] Limited data suggest that the use of a DES after rotational atherectomy has more favorable clinical and angiographic outcomes at 9 months when compared to BMS implantation.[9]

• *Laser atherectomy*: Although initially contraindicated in heavily calcified lesions, more recent innovations allow the operator to vary fluence and pulse repetition settings. The Excimer laser® (Spectranetics Inc., Colorado Springs, CO) can be used as an alternative to RA for plaque modification prior to stent deployment, and it may be of particular advantage in bifurcation lesions, where maintenance of a side branch wire throughout the procedure is desired. Although initial evidence with this technology demonstrated increased procedural success for the delivery of equipment through heavily calcified lesions, subsequent studies into the mechanism of luminal enlargement demonstrated significant deep medial and intimal vascular damage, which led to the decrease in use of this technology with BMSs. Additionally, lack of data surrounding long-term outcomes with laser atherectomy as an adjunct to DESs has led to limited use of the technology during PCI of calcified lesions.[10]

• *Cutting balloons*: Cutting balloons are specially designed balloons aimed at controlling dissection of the coronary plaque during vessel dilation. Once the plaque is "scored" in this fashion, the hoop stress of balloon inflation is decreased, which leads to more consistent expansion of balloons and subsequent stents. The cutting balloon uses lower balloon inflation pressures to achieve a larger lumen gain, which may reduce the incidence of major dissection. It increases the relative contribution of plaque compression to vessel dilation in overall vessel expansion, which may be of particular advantage in the setting of circumferential calcification that significantly inhibits vessel expansion.[11] Two types of cutting balloons are currently available for use in the United States. The Flextome™ (Boston Scientific, Natick, MA) is comprised

Table 7e.2 Adjunctive devices in the treatment of calcified lesions

Device	Author	Year	Endpoint	Lesions (n)	Success	Procedural Complications
RA	MacIsaac[1]	1995	<50% residual without in-hospital death, QWMI, or urgent CABG	1078	94.%	4.1%
RA	Kiesz[2]	1999	Death, emergent CABG, QWMI, NQWMI, TLR within 30 days and at 6 months	146	98.1%	Not reported
CB	Karvouni[3]	2001	Procedural success without death, MI, emergency CABG, or repeat PCI	37	97.3%	2.7%
EL	Fretz[4]	2001	CCS class, CVA, death	7	71.4%	Not reported
EL	Bilodeau[5]	2004	<50% residual without in hospital death, QWMI, NQWMI, or urgent CABG	100	93%	5.3%

RA, rotational atherectomy; CB, cutting balloon; EL, excimer laser; QWMI, Q wave myocardial infarction; NQWMI, non–Q wave myocardial infarction; TLR, target lesion revascularization; CABG, coronary artery bypass graft; MI, myocardial infarction; CCS, Canadian Cardiovascular Society; CVA, cerebrovascular accident.

of three or four microsurgical blades with a 0.005-inch scoring depth, longitudinally mounted on a noncompliant balloon.[12] Randomized data prior to BMS placement suggest improved procedural and long-term outcomes with cutting balloons compared to conventional balloon predilation.[13,14] Studies comparing the Flextome to conventional balloon predilation prior to DES use are ongoing. The Angiosculpt® (Angioscore Inc., Fremont, CA) scoring balloon utilizes three 0.005-inch cylindrical nitinol wires as a scoring device.[15] Nonrandomized and registry data suggest improved stent expansion and long-term clinical outcomes with Angiosculpt scoring compared to either direct stenting or conventional balloon predilation prior to DES placement in complex lesions.[16, 17] The FX Minirail™ Balloon (Abbott Vascular, Abbott Park, IL) is similar in concept to the Angiosculpt; it uses a steerable guidewire that remains external to a semicompliant balloon and a short guidewire lumen distal to the balloon to gain traction across a coronary lesion. By inflating the balloon against these wires, points of highly focal longitudinal stress are introduced at low inflation pressures. Initial studies suggested improved stent expansion, but the balloon is no longer available for use in the United States.[18]

Conclusion

Percutaneous revascularization of heavily calcified coronary stenoses can be extremely difficult and frustrating to the interventional cardiologist. Knowledge of the various types of calcification and their effects on the performance of interventional equipment, along with various special techniques and technologies, can make a significant impact on the success of short- and long-term outcomes following PCI of calcified lesions. A well thought-out strategy with regard to equipment and approach is highly recommended.

Practical Pearls

- Examine extent and distribution of calcium using IVUS.
- Prepare for difficulty with delivery of equipment:
  - Femoral approach
  - Larger (7–8 Fr) guide catheters and extra support shapes
  - Medium support wires
  - "Buddy" wire if needed
- Prepare vessel well prior to stent delivery:
  - Noncompliant balloons
  - Cutting balloon
  - Low threshold for rotational atherectomy
  - Drug-eluting stents

References

1. Mosseri M, Satler LF, Pichard AD, Waksman R. Impact of vessel calcification on outcomes after coronary stenting. *Cardiovasc Revasc Med.* 2005;6:147-153.

2. Tanigawa, J, Barlis P, Di Mario C. Heavily calcified coronary lesions preclude strut apposition despite high pressure balloon dilatation and rotational atherectomy: in vivo demonstration with optical coherence tomography. *Circ J.* 2008;72: 157-160.

3. Albrecht D, Kaspers S, Fussl R, et al. Coronary plaque morphology affects stent deployment: assessment by intracoronary ultrasound. *Cathet Cardiovasc Diagn.* 1996;38:229-235.

4. Tuzcu EM, Berkalp B, DeFranco AC, Ellis SG, et al. The dilemma of diagnosing coronary calcification: angiography versus intravascular ultrasound. *J Am Col Cardiol.* 1996;27:832-838.

5. Mintz GS, Popma JJ, Pichard AD, et al. Patterns of calcification in coronary artery disease. a statistical analysis of intravascular ultrasound and coronary angiography in 1155 lesions. *Circulation.* 1995;91(7):1959-1965.

6. Saland KE, Cigarroa JE, Lange RA, et al. Rotational atherectomy. *Cardiol Rev.* 2000;8(3):174-179.

7. Reisman M. *Guide to rotational atherectomy.* Physician's Press Publishing, Royal Oak, Michigan 1997.

8. Buchbinder M, Fortuna R, Sharma S, et al. Debulking prior to stenting improves acute outcomes: early results from the SPORT trial. *J Am Coll Cardiol.* 2000;35(Suppl A):8A.

9. Khattab AA, Otto A, Hochadel M, et al. Drug-eluting stents versus bare metal stents following rotational atherectomy for heavily calcified coronary lesions: late angiographic and clinical follow-up results. *J Interven Cardiol.* 2007;20:100-106.

10. Mintz GS, Kovach JA, Pichard AD, et al. Intravascular ultrasounding findings after excimer laser coronary angioplasty. *Cathet Cardiovasc Diagn.* 1996;37:113-118.

11. Okura H, Hayase M, Shimodozono S, et al. Mechanisms of acute lumen gain following cutting balloon angioplasty in calcified and noncalcified lesions: an intravascular ultrasound study. *Cathet Cardiovasc Intervent.* 2002;57:429-436.

12. Barath P, Fishbein MC, Vari S, Forrester JS. Cutting balloon: a novel approach to percutaneous angioplasty. *Am J Cardiol.* 1991;68:1249-1252.

13. Ozaki Y, Yamaguchi T, Suzuki T, et al. Impact of cutting balloon angioplasty (CBA) prior to bare metal stenting on restenosis: a prospective randomized multicenter trial comparing CBA with balloon angioplasty (BA) before stenting (REDUCE III). *Circ J.* 2007;71:1-8.

14. Taniuchi M. The WINNER registry, *Catheter Cardiovasc Interv.* 2004;62:36-37.5. Gershony G, Virmani R, Lotan C, et al. A novel angioplasty catheter for the treatment of complex CAD: Angiosculpt. *Am J Cardiol.* 2003;92(6 Suppl)1:166L.

15. Ribamar J, Mintz GS, Carlier S, et al. Nonrandomized comparison of coronary stenting under intravascular ultrasound guidance of direct stenting without predilatation versus conventional predilatation with a semi-compliant balloon versus predilation with a new scoring balloon. *Am J Cardiol.* 2007;100(5):A1-A18.

16. Grenadier E, Kerner A, Gershony G, et al. Optimizing plaque modification in complex lesions utilizing the AngioSculpt device: acute and long term results from a large two-center registry. *Am J Cardiol.* 2008;102(8) Suppl 1:53I-54I.

17. Viterella G, Sangiorgi G, Koronowski R, et al. FX MiniRAIL catheter usage for treatment of de novo complex coronary lesions: results from the "OFFAR." *J Interv Cardiol.* 2006;19(3):250-257.

Chapter 7f

Bifurcation Lesions

Jose G. Diez and James M. Wilson

Bifurcation lesions constitute up to 20% of all coronary lesions treated with percutaneous coronary intervention (PCI).[1] Treating bifurcation lesions is challenging because of the threats of side-branch closure, early thrombosis, and especially restenosis. The presence of one or more bifurcation lesions strongly influences the decision whether to refer the patient for coronary artery bypass graft (CABG) surgery.[2]

Angioplasty of bifurcation lesions is associated with higher-than-normal complication rates because of ineffective lumen expansion, a consequence of plaque shift (longitudinal displacement of plaque) and lesion recoil. Stenting reduces recoil, thus achieving a larger effective lumen. Unfortunately, exaggerated plaque shift caused by stenting the main branch may compromise side branches.

One option for bifurcation PCI with stents is simply treating the main branch with provisional angioplasty or stenting of the side branch. Another option is stenting both the main branch and side branch (Figs. 7f.1 and 7f.2). In cases in which both the main vessel and the side branch are stented, reported incidences of major adverse events range up to 9%.[3] Thus, the simpler approach—stenting the main branch and provisionally stenting the side branch—is currently used in most instances. This technique is associated with a 98% angiographic success rate in both branches. Two stents are used in 30%–35% of cases, and final "kissing" balloon inflation is performed in more than 95% of cases. The in-hospital rate of major adverse cardiac events (MACEs) has been reported to be around 5%, and the 7-month target-vessel revascularization rate (TVR) has been estimated at 13%.[4]

Routine side-branch stent implantation has been compared to provisional side-branch stenting with either the T-stent or the crush technique. Reintervention rates are reportedly no different at 6 months (5.0% vs 7.9%; p = 0.39) and 1 year (8.9% vs 10.9%; p = NS).[5] A similar trial of the crush technique alone versus provisional side-branch stenting arrived at similar conclusions. Still, both groups had high rates of MACE (15.8% in the crush group vs. 15% in the provisional-stenting group, p = NS).[6]

Provisional side-branch stenting is associated with a lower incidence of adverse outcomes at 1 year when drug-eluting stents (DESs) are used (death,

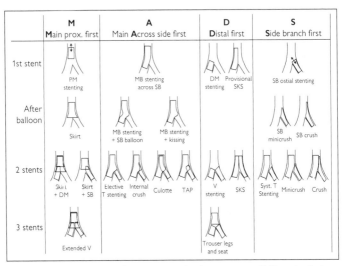

Figure 7f.1 The MADS classification system for the treatment of bifurcation lesions. Reprinted from Legrand V, et al. Percutaneous coronary intervention of bifurcation lesions: state-of-the-art. Insights from the second meeting of the European Bifurcation Club. *EurInterv.* 2007; 3:44-49, with permission of the publisher (Europa Edition).

Figure 7f.2 The MADS classification scheme for "inverted" treatment techniques. Reprinted from Legrand V, et al. Percutaneous coronary intervention of bifurcation lesions: state-of-the-art. Insights from the second meeting of the European Bifurcation Club. *EurInterv.* 2007; 3:44-49, with permission of the publisher (Europa Edition).

2.4%; myocardial infarction, 4.0%; revascularization, 5.6%) than when bare metal stents (BMS) are used.[7] Therefore, provisional stenting with DESs appears to be both the safest and the most effective option.

Planning and Risk Assessment

To determine the technique most likely to be effective for a particular type of bifurcation lesion, various classification schemes have been developed that are based on angiographic morphology.[8] However, fractional flow reserve (FFR) may be more accurate than angiography in identifying side-branch lesions that have significant physiologic effects and that therefore require additional attention (see Chapter 6).[9]

The first step in approaching a bifurcation lesion is discovering the impact of the lesion's angiographic morphology and the size of the side branch. Generally, one should attempt to preserve any at-risk side branch of greater than 2.0 mm in diameter. If the side branch is smaller than 2.0 mm, the risk of short- or long-term failure of the intervention in the main branch probably exceeds the potential benefit of attempting to preserve the small side branch (Fig. 7f.3).

The anatomic descriptive classification systems provide useful information regarding the short- and long-term risk of failure. It may be wisest to adopt a combination of simple schemes that includes the useful subscripts describing angulation, calcification, or left main coronary artery involvement.[8] Angulation and calcification may both influence the likelihood that cutting-balloon or rotational atherectomy will be needed to maximize the chances of success if provisional side-branch stent implantation is necessary.[10,11]

The European "Bifurcation Club" adopted the Medina classification (Fig. 7f.4), in which a 0 indicates no disease and a 1 indicates significant disease in any of three locations: proximal, distal, and side branch.[12] Lesion angulation, which then defines the most appropriate approach, is described with a similarly easy classification scheme (MADS: main, across, distal, side).[13]

Equipment

Equipment choices are a function of aortic and coronary anatomy, as well as lesion characteristics. The choice of guide is determined by the angulation proximal to the lesion, the angulation of the lesion, and the severity of calcification. Generally, once you have determined the minimum guide support that you suspect will be successful, step it up one notch. If final dilation with a kissing balloon is anticipated, ensure that the inner lumen (7 or 8 Fr) will accommodate two balloons. Guiding-catheter choice may be the key to success, and in a bifurcation case, it is a choice that you cannot take back.

The choice of wires is a function of the technique to be used. If the main branch is the principal target, any floppy-tipped wire is appropriate. For the side branch, a hydrophilic wire should be used in anticipation of the possibility of

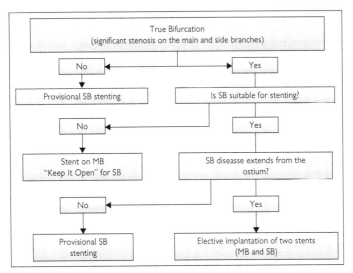

Figure 7f.3 An algorithm for the treatment of bifurcation lesions. Reprinted from Latib A, Colombo A. Bifurcation disease: what do we know, what should we do? *JACC Cardiovasc Interv.* 2008;1(3):218-226, with permission of the publisher (Elsevier).

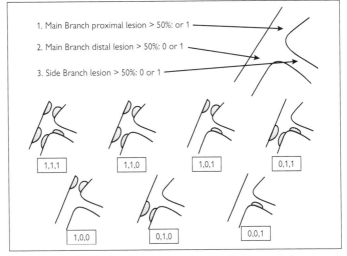

Figure 7f.4 An illustration of the Medina classification of bifurcation lesions. Reprinted from Latib A, Colombo A. Bifurcation disease: what do we know, what should we do? *JACC Cardiovasc Interv.* 2008;1(3):218-226, with permission of the publisher (Elsevier).

trapping the wire beneath the main-branch stent, which allows easy identification of the site of entry to the side branch. If the side branch is to be stented first, then a floppy-tipped wire is used there, and the hydrophilic wire is used in the main branch. Recrossing into a vessel through the side struts is more easily accomplished with a hydrophilic wire.

With respect to stent choices, stent designs differ in the maximum diameter that can be achieved by side-strut dilation. Therefore, the size of the side branch (or main branch) should be the most important determinant of stent choice.

Techniques

For almost all bifurcation lesions with a significant side branch, both vessels should be wired. When it is likely that the bifurcation lesion endangers the side branch, or if there is ostial or more extensive side-branch disease (Medina 1.1.1, 1.0.1, 0.1.1), both branches are alternately predilated.

The initial plan is to implant the main-branch stent so as to leave the side-branch wire "jailed." A third wire is then advanced into the side branch, and the jailed wire is used as a guide to the location of the side-branch ostium. After the wire is successfully placed in the side branch, the jailed wire may be removed. After predilation through the stent struts, final kissing-balloon postdilation is performed. In the event that residual stenosis of greater 75% remains in the side branch, a second stent may be deployed (T-technique) in the nonstented side branch. Avoid excessively stretching the proximal left main artery when both balloons are inflated simultaneously (Table 7f.1).

If significant extra-ostial disease is present within the side branch, or if occlusive or near-occlusive dissection of the side branch results from predilation, the side branch should be stented first, and only secondary attention should be paid to the distal main branch.

Alternative Techniques

In the "classical crush" technique, a stent is positioned in the side branch with about one-third of its length protruding into the main branch. Another stent is positioned in the main branch (covering the proximal and distal segments of the lesion and the ostium of the side branch). The side-branch stent is deployed, and if there is no downstream dissection, the side-branch balloon and wire are removed. The main-branch stent is then deployed, crushing the portion of the side-branch stent lying in the main branch. The side branch is rewired, and postdilation kissing-balloon angioplasty is done.

In the "mini-crush" technique, the side-branch stent is slightly retracted into the main vessel, and a balloon is used to crush the side-branch stent rather than the main-branch stent. This procedure is followed by the jailed wire technique, then kissing-balloon angioplasty.

Table 7f.1 Stepwise approach

1. Wire all side-branches ≥2 mm in diameter, crossing the most difficult part of the lesion first.

2. Plan on provisional side-branch treatment if possible and provisional side-branch stenting if side-branch treatment is necessary. A planned, modified Y-technique (stenting the distal main branch and side branch only) may be considered if the proximal main segment is completely normal. Consider IVUS or FFR to guide your decision.

3. For bifurcation lesions with involvement of the side-branch ostium, predilate both the side-branch and the main branch.

4. For provisional side-branch treatment, decide whether to predilate the side branch after the main branch is predilated.

5. Stent the main branch first unless there is potential abrupt closure of the side branch or the angle of the side branch remains ≥90 degrees after wiring and side-branch stent treatment is deemed necessary.

6. "Jail" the side-branch wire with the main-branch stent.

7. Obtain side-branch wire access via stent side struts, using the original side-branch wire as a guide.

8. Remove the original side-branch wire and balloon the origin of the side branch.

9. If the side-branch result is acceptable, ≤75% stenosis with TIMI 3 flow, perform final kissing-balloon postdilation, using high-pressure inflation in the main branch only.

10. Stent the side branch if the residual stenosis is ≤75% or < TIMI 3 flow, using the T-technique.

11. End with kissing-balloon postdilation, alternately using high-pressure inflation in either branch, ending with the main branch. Each balloon should be noncompliant and sized to the distal vessel into which it will be inserted.

IVUS, intravascular ultrasound; FFR, fractional flow reserve.

Two-Stent Approach to Bifurcation Lesions

A number of two-stent approaches are currently used in practice. These include T-stenting, V-stenting, the crush technique, and the culotte technique. The T-stenting technique involves positioning a stent at the ostium of the side branch, being careful to avoid stent protrusion into the main vessel. Subsequently, a second stent is deployed in the main vessel and final kissing balloon angioplasty is performed. V-stenting technique refers to delivery and implantation of two stents simultaneously. For this, one stent is advanced in the main vessel and the other in the side branch, with the proximal extent of both stents touching and forming a small carina. For the crush technique, stents are placed in the main vessel and the side branch, with the stent in the main vessel placed more proximally than the latter. The stent of the side branch is deployed, followed by deployment in the main vessel, which flattens/crushes the protruding cells of the side-branch stent. Final kissing balloon inflation should be performed to redilate the stent in the side branch. For the culotte technique, a stent is deployed across the smaller, more angulated branch, typically the side branch. Then the nonstented branch is rewired through the struts of the stent and dilated. A second stent is then deployed in the nonstented branch, usually the main vessel. Final kissing

Table 7f.2 Practical pearls
• Regarding bifurcation stenting "You can do it, but . . . Should you do it?"
• Consider the side branch: Does it need protection, treatment, a stent, or a combination of these?
• If you get fancy, you get complications.
• Consider rotational atherectomy or cutting-balloon predilation (plaque modification).
• Consider using IVUS, FFR, or both to guide therapy.
• Give it a "kiss" before you leave.
IVUS, intravascular ultrasound; FFR, fractional flow reserve.

balloon inflation is then performed. The preferred strategy depends on operator experience with each technique, with minimal comparative data available.

Special Issues

- Bifurcation intervention demands an appropriate balance among the clinical justification for the intervention (i.e., the expected benefit), the need to achieve an optimal result, the procedural risk, and the long-term outcome (Table 7f.2).
- Several stents specifically designed for coronary bifurcation lesions are being investigated.[14]

Conclusion

The best percutaneous treatment of bifurcation lesions has not been established. Treating bifurcation lesions is challenging because of the threats of side-branch closure, early thrombosis, and especially restenosis. Based on available data, the strategy of stenting the main vessel with provisional side-branch stenting is the currently favored approach, although there are situations in which a two-stent strategy should be considered, such as the presence of a large side branch that supplies a significant area of myocardium.

Practical Pearls

- Characterize the bifurcation anatomy to determine whether side-branch treatment is necessary, and assess the potential difficulty of this procedure by using the Medina classification, lesion angulation, and severity of calcification.
- Never skimp on guide support for the catheter.
- Wire both vessels if the side branch is 2 mm or more in diameter.
- Keep it simple. Treat the main branch only, if possible, and stent the side branch only when necessary.
- Finish with kissing-balloon dilation.

References

1. Al Suwaidi J, Yeh W, Cohen HA, Detre KM, Williams DO, Holmes DR, Jr. Immediate and one-year outcome in patients with coronary bifurcation lesions in the modern era (NHLBI dynamic registry). Am J Cardiol. 2001;87(10):1139-1144.

2. Serruys PW, Morice MC, Kappetein AP, et al. Percutaneous coronary intervention versus coronary-artery bypass grafting for severe coronary artery disease. N Engl J Med. 2009;360(10):961-972.

3. Fischman DL, Savage MP, Leon MB, et al. Fate of lesion-related side branches after coronary artery stenting. J Am Coll Cardiol. 1993;22(6):1641-1646.

4. Lefevre T, Louvard Y, Morice MC, Loubeyre C, Piechaud JF, Dumas P. Stenting of bifurcation lesions: a rational approach. J Interv Cardiol. 2001;14(6):573-585.

5. Ferenc M, Gick M, Kienzle RP, et al. Randomized trial on routine vs. provisional T-stenting in the treatment of de novo coronary bifurcation lesions. Eur Heart J. 2008;29(23):2859-2867.

6. Colombo A, Bramucci E, Sacca S, et al. Randomized study of the crush technique versus provisional side-branch stenting in true coronary bifurcations: the CACTUS (Coronary Bifurcations: Application of the Crushing Technique Using Sirolimus-Eluting Stents) Study. Circulation. 2009;119(1):71-78.

7. Suzuki N, Angiolillo DJ, Tannenbaum MA, et al. Strategies for drug-eluting stent treatment of bifurcation coronary artery disease in the United States: insights from the e-Cypher S.T.L.L.R. trial. Catheter Cardiovasc Interv. 2009;73(7):890-897.

8. Movahed MR, Kern K, Thai H, Ebrahimi R, Friedman M, Slepian M. Coronary artery bifurcation lesions: a review and update on classification and interventional techniques. Cardiovasc Revasc Med. 2008;9(4):263-268.

9. Koo BK, Park KW, Kang HJ, et al. Physiological evaluation of the provisional side-branch intervention strategy for bifurcation lesions using fractional flow reserve. Eur Heart J. 2008;29(6):726-732.

10. Takebayashi H, Haruta S, Kohno H, et al. Immediate and 3-month follow-up outcome after cutting balloon angioplasty for bifurcation lesions. J Interv Cardiol. 2004;17(1):1-7.

11. Nageh T, Kulkarni NM, Thomas MR. High-speed rotational atherectomy in the treatment of bifurcation-type coronary lesions. Cardiology. 2001;95(4):198-205.

12. Legrand V, Thomas M, Zelisko M, et al. Percutaneous coronary intervention of bifurcation lesions: state of the art. Insights from the second meeting of the European Bifurcation Club. EuroIntervention. 2007;3:44-49.

13. Stankovic G, Darremont O, Ferenc M, et al. Percutaneous coronary intervention for bifurcation lesions: 2008 consensus document from the fourth meeting of the European Bifurcation Club. EuroIntervention. 2009;5:39-49.

14. Verheye S, Agostoni P, Dubois CL, et al. 9-month clinical, angiographic, and intravascular ultrasound results of a prospective evaluation of the Axxess self-expanding biolimus A9-eluting stent in coronary bifurcation lesions: the DIVERGE (Drug-Eluting Stent Intervention for Treating Side Branches Effectively) study. J Am Coll Cardiol. 2009;53(12):1031-1039.

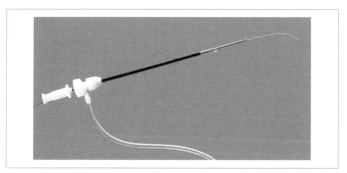

Figure 3.1 **Cook micropuncture kit**. This radial artery access kit utilizes a 21-gauge needle for arterial access, over which a 0.018-inch nitinol wire is advanced. The outer surface of the introducer and the distal tip of the inner dilator are coated with AQ® hydrophilic coating. Depending on the manufacturer, sheaths are available in long (23 cm), standard (13 cm), and short (7 cm) lengths.

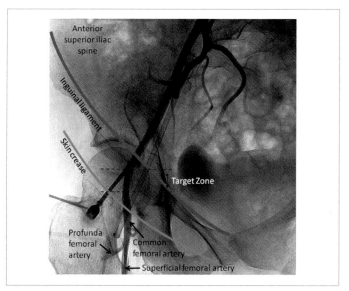

Figure 3.3 Femoral arterial access using fluoroscopic landmarks.

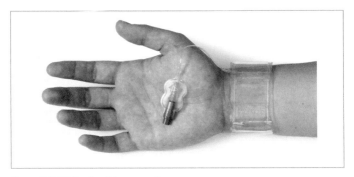

Figure 3.9 **TR Band radial compression system.**

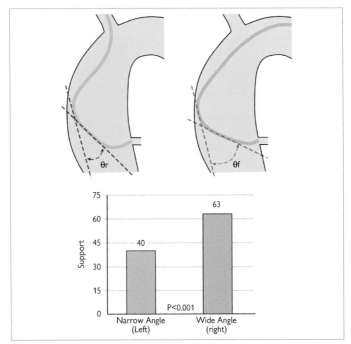

Figure 4.1 **Importance of secondary curve and aortic wall angle in support.** Ikari et al.[2] performed elegant experiments to analyze the physics of support provided by guiding catheters. Their findings confirmed the clinical experience that support is affected by two aortic root factors: (1) the angle the catheter makes with the contralateral aortic wall, and (2) the length of the contact area of the catheter against the contralateral wall. This highlights the importance of considering aortic root dimensions in determining the likely amount of support provided by the guiding catheter. θ refers to angle between catheter and contralateral wall; r, radial access; f, femoral access. Reprinted from Ikari Y, Nagaoka M, Kim JY, Morino Y, Tanabe T. The physics of guiding catheters for the left coronary artery in transfemoral and transradial interventions. *J Invas Cardiol.* 2005;17:636-641, with permission of the publisher (HMP Communications).

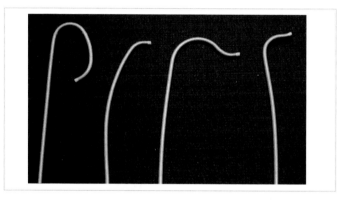

Figure 4.7 **Commonly used angioplasty guide catheters for the native coronary arteries.** From left to right, the Judkins left (JL) coronary curve, the Judkins right (JR) curve, the Amplatz left (AL) coronary curve, and the Amplatz right (AR) coronary curve. Reprinted from Holmes DR, Mathew V. *Atlas of interventional cardiology*, 2nd ed. Philadelphia: Current Medicine, Inc., 2003, with permission of the publisher (Current Medicine Group LLC).

Table 4.5 Features of common guiding catheters

Name		Curvature	Size (cm)	Advantages	Disadvantages
Judkins Left (JL)		1° curve: 90 degrees 2° curve: 180 degrees	Determined by length of arm between 1° and 2° curves: JL3.5, JL4, JL5, JL6	• Adequate for straightforward LAD PCI cases • May be best choice in ostial lesions	• Sharp primary curve may limit coaxial alignment in many cases • Poor support in complex LCX cases
Judkins Right (JR)		1° curve: 90 degrees 2° curve: 30 degrees	Determined by length of secondary curve: JR3.5, JR4, JR5, JR6	• Adequate for simple RCA PCI cases	Primary curve limits coaxial engagement in anterior RCA and superiorly RCA take-off
Amplatz Left (AL)	Amplatz Right (AR)	1° curve: tapered tip perpendicular to secondary curve 2° curve: pre-shaped half circle	Determined by length of secondary curve: AL1-AL3, AR1-AR3	• Provides excellent support for most complex PCI • Appropriate for LCX lesion • Useful in cases where JL/JR guides unable to provide adequate support	May not be useful and is not recommended for ostial lesions
Extra Back-Up (XB)		Straight tip with long circular curve	Determined by length of secondary curve: XB3.0, XB 3.5, XB4.0	• Provides excellent support due to long circular curve laying against contralateral aortic wall • Commonly used in most labs as workforce guide for left coronary interventions	May not be appropriate for very short left main
Multipurpose (MPA)		Straight with single minor bend at tip (primary curve)		Can be used for hard to engage grafts	Not used commonly

PCI, percutaneous coronary intervention; LAD, left anterior descending; LCX, left circumflex; RCA, right coronary artery.

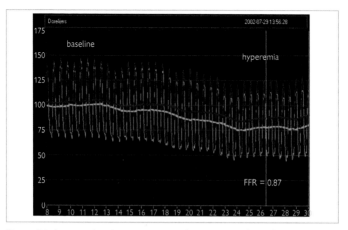

Figure 6.1 A screen shot demonstrating simultaneous recordings of aortic pressure and post-stenotic arterial pressure used to calculate fractional flow reserve (FFR). In this case, the FFR was 0.87 at maximal hyperemia, indicating a non–flow limiting stenosis.

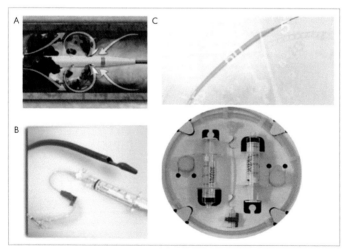

Figure 7a.2 Thrombectomy devices. (A) Different thrombectomy devices currently used in ST elevation myocardial infarction (STEMI) intervention. AngioJet thrombectomy device. (B) Different thrombectomy devices currently used in ST elevation myocardial infarction (STEMI) intervention. Pronto extraction catheter. (C) Different thrombectomy devices currently used in ST elevation myocardial infarction (STEMI) intervention. Export manual aspiration catheter.

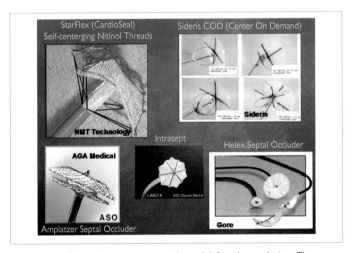

Figure 12a.1 **Selected percutaneous atrial septal defect closure devices.** The manufacturers are imprinted on the pictures.

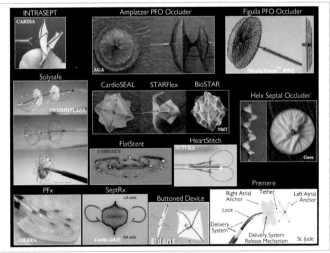

Figure 12a.2 **Selected percutaneous patent foramen ovale closure devices.** The manufacturers are imprinted on the pictures.

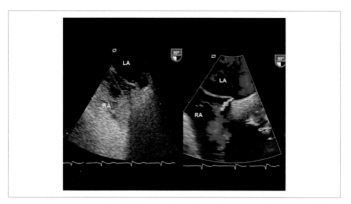

Figure 12a.4 **Transesophageal echocardiography proving a patent foramen ovale** by passage of aerated saline appearing as bubbles (*left*) and as a Doppler shunt (*right*) through a patent foramen ovale after a Valsalva maneuver. Patency of the foramen ovale can be semiquantitatively assessed by counting the number of bubbles in the left atrium on a still frame: small shunt (0–5 bubbles), moderate shunt (6–20 bubbles), large shunt (>20 bubbles). LA, left atrium; RA, right atrium.

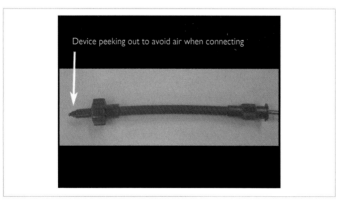

Figure 12a.8 **Placement of an Amplatzer Septal Occluder.** Step 4: Device within the loader ready for connection with the delivery sheath.

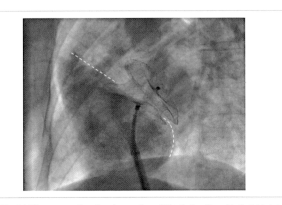

Figure 12a.14 **Placement of an Amplatzer Septal Occluder.** Step 10: A right atrial contrast angiogram delineates the atrial septum (*dashed lines*). The device should be visualized in perfect profile without any disk overlap. The device is then released.

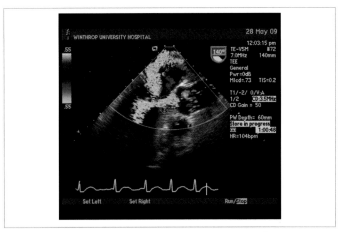

Figure 12b.2 **Mitral regurgitation.** Transesophageal echocardiography is necessary in patients with moderate to severe mitral regurgitation, in order to assess etiology of mitral regurgitation (MR). Mitral regurgitation due to hypertrophic obstructive cardiomyopathy and systolic anterior motion of the mitral valve results in posteriorly directed MR. Turbulence to flow in the outflow tract that divides into two separate jets (one into the aorta and the other posteriorly directed into the left atrium) results in the classic "Y" sign, indicating that MR is solely related to hypertrophic obstructive cardiomyopathy and is likely to respond to septal reduction therapy.

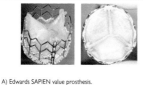

A) Edwards SAPIEN value prosthesis.
   Balloon-expandable
   Stented prosthesis
   Stainless steel tubular frame
   Tri-leaflet bovine pericardial tissue value
   (sutured within frame)
   Lengthened fabric sealing cuff.

B) SAPIEN XT value prosthesis.
   Balloon-expandable
   Stented prosthesis
   Cobalt-chromium frame (thinner struts)
   Tri-leaflet bovine pericardial tissue value
   (sutured within frame)
   Lengthened fabric sealing cuff.

Figure 12c.2 **Edwards valve prostheses.**

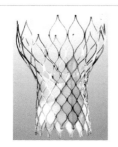 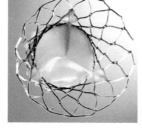

Self-expanding
50-mm-long nitinol stent
Three bovine pericardial leaflets (mounted and sutured within the frame)
Supra-annular value function
Intra-annular implantation
Sealing skirt

Figure 12c.3 **CoreValve prosthesis.**

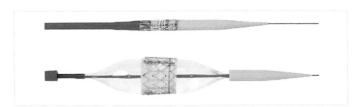

Figure 12c.4 RetroFlex2 delivery system for Edwards prostheses.

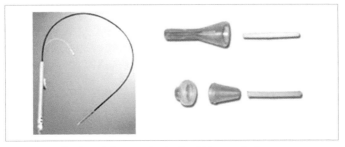

Figure 12c.5 Revalving delivery system for CoreValve prosthesis.

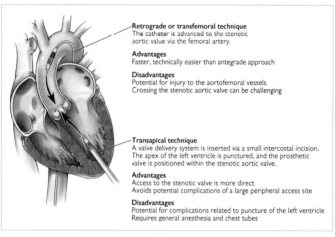

Retrograde or transfemoral technique
The catheter is advanced to the stenotic aortic value via the femoral artery.

Advantages
Faster, technically easier than antegrade approach

Disadvantages
Potential for injury to the aortofemoral vessels
Crossing the stenotic aortic valve can be challenging

Transapical technique
A valve delivery system is inserted via a small intercostal incision. The apex of the left ventricle is punctured, and the prosthetic valve is positioned within the stenotic aortic valve.

Advantages
Access to the stenotic valve is more direct
Avoids potential complications of a large peripheral access site

Disadvantages
Potential for complications related to puncture of the left ventricle
Requires general anesthesia and chest tubes

Figure 12c.6 Retrograde and transapical approaches. From Singh IM, Shishehbor MH, Christofferson RD, Tuzcu EM, Kapadia SR. Percutaneous treatment of aortic valve stenosis. *Cleve Clin J Med.* 2008;75(11):805-812, with permission of the publisher (Cleveland Clinic Center for Medical Art & Photography).

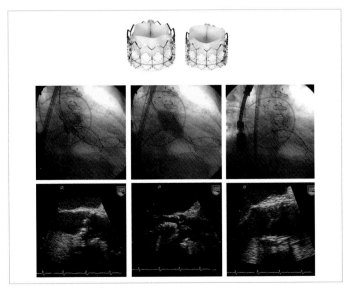

Figure 12c.7 **Edwards SAPIEN deployment.**

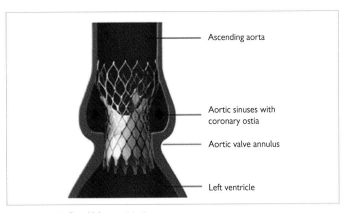

Ascending aorta

Aortic sinuses with coronary ostia

Aortic valve annulus

Left ventricle

Figure 12c.10 **CoreValve positioning.**

Chapter 7g

Left Internal Mammary Artery Graft Lesions

Carl Dragstedt

The widespread use of left internal mammary arteries (LIMAs) as coronary artery bypass conduits ushered in dramatic improvements in outcomes when compared with saphenous vein aortocoronary bypass grafts.[1] The patency rate for internal mammary arteries at 10 years is approximately 85%, as opposed to a reverse saphenous vein graft rate of 61% over the same time period.[2] Radial artery grafts portend an even poorer prognostic patency rate at 2 years, approximately 51%.[3] Pathophysiologically, LIMAs offer distinct advantages over saphenous vein or radial artery conduits post-coronary artery bypass grafting (CABG); they tend to have lower rates of atherosclerosis, and late graft loss is generally due to fibrointimal hyperplasia and proliferation as opposed to progressive atherosclerotic disease (Table 7g.1).[4] Despite their prevalent usage, LIMA graft failure or obstruction rarely occurs. Although found with a low incidence, angiographic and functionally significant lesions involving IMAs are most often detected at distal graft-target anastomoses, which usually occur within the first few months after surgery. Lesions may also occur in downstream native vessels supplied by the graft, whereas obstructive lesions within the body of the LIMA are exceedingly rare. Consequently, clinical data are not robust regarding the optimal approach to LIMA lesions with regards to technical, adjunctive pharmacologic, and patient-specific aspects. Long-term outcome data are particularly scarce, and the paucity of data is even greater in the current stent era.

Results of Internal Mammary Artery Graft Interventions

Patient Management: Preprocedural Considerations

As with all angiographic interpretations, it is imperative to determine the appropriateness of all therapeutic options, ranging from intensified medical therapy alone to percutaneous versus surgical revascularization. Verifying the presence of clinical indicators, including angina, ischemia, or infarction, are key determinants that favor mechanical revascularization, yet unlike native coronary

Table 7g.1 Results of internal mammary artery graft interventions

Year	Study	No. of Patients	Success (%)
1991	Dimas et al.[5]	31	90
1991	Shimshak et al.[6]	86	94
1992	Sketch et al.[7]	14	93
1995	Hearne et al.[8]	68	88
1995	Najm et al.[9]	34	91
1995	Ishizaka et al.[10]	46	74
2000	Mann et al.[11]	10	100
2000	Gruberg et al.[12]	174	97
2001	Sharma et al.[13]	280	92
2001	Roffi et al.[14]	225	87

anatomy, several unique aspects of LIMAs and the distal bypassed anatomy should be considered prior to proceeding.

Coronary lesions downstream of the anastomosis *may* be accessible through the native coronary anatomy, thereby obviating the technical challenges of navigating through the bypass conduit, which is frequently quite tortuous (Fig. 7g.1). If feasible, this approach should be considered for two principal reasons. First, negotiating the guide catheter into the ostium of the IMA requires one or more acute turns to ensure adequate coaxial positioning with optimal back support. Second, the distance from access site and through the LIMA may limit the passage of the guidewire, angioplasty balloon, and stent-delivery system. This issue is usually addressed with a 90-cm guide. Moreover, the extreme tortuosity frequently encountered in LIMAs further increases the risk of vessel pseudostenosis, dissection, or perforation. The use of fractional flow reserve or intravascular ultrasound has not been well studied in the LIMA.

Key patient-specific factors also warrant attention. Awareness of renal dysfunction is critical. The diagnostic catheterization may already necessitate higher contrast volumes to allow native and graft angiography, and graft intervention may result in a greater increase in contrast load. Outside of the acute coronary syndromes, it is reasonable to delay interventions until after diagnostic angiography, thereby monitoring and allowing time for renal recovery. This approach allows for temporal resolution of any underlying renal dysfunction and for the readministration of contrast-induced nephropathy prophylaxis prior to intervention. If percutaneous intervention is planned, it is essential to have an understanding of the patient's bleeding risk and whether any noncardiac procedures are planned, as both of these may dictate stent type, hence the minimum duration of dual antiplatelet therapy.

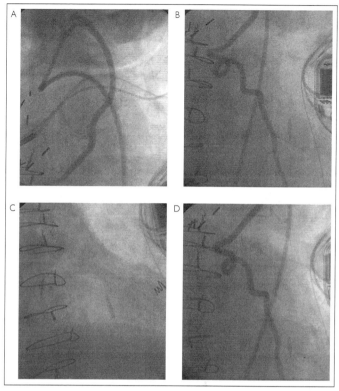

Figure 7g.1 (A) Engagement of the left internal mammary artery (LIMA) with a 7 Fr 90 cm Raabe sheath and a 6 Fr VB1 guide catheter. (B) Extreme vessel tortuosity, with high-grade stenosis at anastomosis. (C) Prowater wire and balloon angioplasty. Even with the support offered from the Raabe guiding sheath, a stent was unable to be delivered. (D) Final angiographic result. (Courtesy of RD Anderson.)

Management of the Patient: Procedural Considerations

Given the proclivity of LIMA angiography to cause patient chest wall discomfort, we recommend the use of nonionic contrast medium for LIMA interventions, particularly given the likelihood of repeated injections in multiple orthogonal views. Femoral arterial access generally allows engagement of the LIMA. In the event of difficult engagement or excessive total distance from point of access to distal targets, an ipsilateral brachial or radial approach is recommended.

The choice of guiding catheter often is determined based on the anatomy revealed at the time of diagnostic catheterization. An IMA or VB1 guide may offer both better anatomic alignment as well as stable positioning. Coaxial engagement of the LIMA ostium allows for optimal stability and support to facilitate equipment passage. Moreover, it minimizes the risk of repeated engagements/disengagements, and potentially reduces the risk of subclavian or ostial LIMA dissection.

Standard guidewires are generally acceptable to use when crossing the LIMA and distal vasculature. However, due to frequent tortuosity, we generally recommend a hydrophilic, flexible guidewire, understanding that stability and support may be suboptimal with their usage. Pseudolesions or wire bias may be encountered, which are a function of vessel tortuosity and wire stiffness. We advocate the use of a compliant angioplasty balloon, both to allow greater flexibility and to facilitate removal following inflation within a potentially tortuous and dissection-prone vessel segment. Although there is no established benefit to drug-eluting stents (DESs) over bare metal stents (BMSs), the use of DESs may be appropriate in certain clinical situations, such as in diabetics, long lesions, and those at highest risk of restenosis.[15]

Adjunctive pharmacotherapy involving LIMA graft interventions should be dictated by the clinical indication. Ideally, up-front dual antiplatelet therapy with aspirin and clopidogrel is recommended for all interventions, both for percutaneous transluminal coronary angioplasty (PTCA) and for percutaneous coronary intervention (PCI), and it should be continued based on the nature of the stent deployed. Systemic anticoagulation should be administered once the decision to proceed with intervention has been made and before guidewire passage. Although the benefit of glycoprotein IIb/IIIa inhibitors (GPIs) in saphenous vein graft interventions has not been demonstrated,[16] their use in LIMA graft interventions has neither been validated nor refuted in terms of benefit. We advocate provisional GPI usage rather than routine upstream usage, including in non-ST segment elevation acute coronary syndromes.

Conclusion

Left IMA graft lesions present a particularly challenging technical subset of those undergoing PCI. Regardless of lesion location, engagement and navigation of the LIMA commands awareness of both LIMA and native vessel anatomy to allow for optimal access, equipment selection, and limitation of iatrogenic trauma during the procedure.

Practical Pearls

- Consider native vessel approach if possible to traverse distal target.
- Consider ipsilateral arm access in presence of difficult engagement or inadequate length.
- A 90-cm sheath offers enhanced support and facilitates equipment passage.
- Flexible, hydrophilic guidewires allow easier navigation through tortuous vessels.
- Compliant balloons allow greater flexibility and ease of passage and removal.
- Consider the use of DESs in those at highest risk of restenosis.

References

1. Loop FD, Lytle BW, Cosgrove DM et al. Influence of the internal mammary artery graft on 10-year survival and other cardiac events. *N Engl J Med.* 1986;314:1-6.

2. Goldman S, Zadina K, Moritz T, et al. Long-term patency of saphenous vein and left internal mammary artery grafts after coronary artery bypass surgery: results from a Department of Veterans Affairs Cooperative Study. *J Am Coll Cardiol.* 2004;44(11):2149-2156.

3. Khot UN, Friedman DT, Pettersson G, et al. Radial artery bypass grafts have an increased occurrence of angiographically severe stenosis and occlusion compared with left internal mammary arteries and saphenous vein grafts. *Circulation.* 2004;109(17):2086-2091.

4. Shelton ME, Forman MB, Virmani R, et al. A comparison of morphologic and angiographic findings in long-term internal mammary artery and saphenous vein bypass grafts. *J Am Coll Cardiol.* 1988;11(2):297-307.

5. Dimas AP, Arora RR, Whitlow PL, et al. Percutaneous transluminal angioplasty involving internal mammary artery grafts. *Am Heart J.* 1991;122(2):423-429.

6. Shimshak TM, Rutherford BD, McConahay DR, et al. PTCA of internal mammary artery (IMA) grafts: Procedural results and late follow-up. *Circulation.* 1991;84(Suppl II):II-590.

7. Sketch MH Jr., Quigley PJ, Perez JA, et al. Angiographic follow-up after internal mammary artery graft angioplasty. *Am J Cardiol.* 1992;70(3):401-403.

8. Hearne SE, Wilson JS, Harrington J et al. Angiographic and clinical follow-up after internal mammary artery graft angioplasty: a 9-year experience. *J Am Coll Cardiol.* 1995;25(Suppl A):139A.

9. Najm HK, Leddy D, Hendry PJ, et al. Postoperative symptomatic internal thoracic artery stenosis and successful treatment with PTCA. *Ann Thorac Surg.* 1995;59(2):323-326.

10. Ishizaka N, Ishizaka Y, Ikari Y, et al. Initial and subsequent angiographic outcome of percutaneous transluminal angioplasty performed on internal mammary artery grafts. *Br Heart J.* 1995;74(6):615-619.

11. Mann T, Cubeddu G, Schneider J, et al. Left internal mammary artery intervention: the left radial approach with a new guide catheter. *J Invasive Cardiol.* 2000;12(6):298-302.

12. Gruberg L, Dangas G, Mehran R, et al. Percutaneous revascularization of the internal mammary artery graft: short- and long-term outcomes. *J Am Coll Cardiol.* 200015;35(4):944-948.

13. Sharma A, McGlynn S, Pinnnow E, et al. Internal mammary artery intervention: to stent or not to stent? A study of 280 patients. *Circulation.* 2001;104(Suppl II):II-705.

14. Roffi M, Mukherjee D, Chew DP, et al. Procedural success and outcomes of percutaneous coronary interventions on arterial bypass grafts. *Circulation.* 2001;104(Suppl II):II-776.

15. Buch AN, Xue Z, Gevorkian NN, et al. Comparison of outcomes between bare metal stents and drug-eluting stents for percutaneous revascularization of internal mammary grafts. *Am J Cardiol.* 2006;98(6):722-724. Epub 2006 Jul 21.

16. Roffi M, Mukherjee D, Chew DP, et al. Lack of benefit from intravenous platelet glycoprotein IIb/IIIa receptor inhibition as adjunctive treatment for percutaneous interventions of aortocoronary bypass grafts: a pooled analysis of five randomized clinical trials. *Circulation.* 2002;106(24):3063-3037.

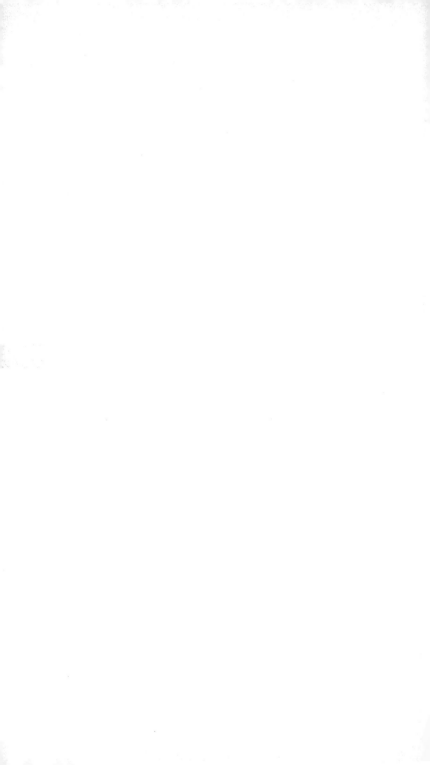

Chapter 7h

Left Main Coronary Interventions

Hussam Hamdalla

Despite the constant and steady improvement in procedural safety and long-term lesion outcomes for percutaneous coronary intervention (PCI), the unprotected left main (LM) has remained mostly the province of cardiac surgery. The survival advantage of coronary artery bypass graft (CABG) surgery compared to medical management has made it the standard of care since the 1970s. Technical advances in PCI and stent technology have emboldened the interventional cardiology community to test the feasibility of and document the procedural results for stenting the left main coronary artery. Initial short- and mid-term results with percutaneous revascularization were disappointing[1]; however, this outcome was revamped with the introduction of newer stents. Drug-eluting stents (DESs) represented a large leap forward in the PCI arena. However, despite the progress we have made in tackling this lesion, we still lack long-term data. Furthermore, the left main poses a technical challenge to the interventional cardiologist because of its anatomical complexity compared to the other coronary arteries.

Patient Management

Since surgical revascularization remains the standard of care for LM disease, the majority of patients referred for PCI are high-risk patients rejected for surgery for an array of different reasons. They are more likely to have comorbidities, including poor left ventricular (LV) function, congestive heart failure, renal failure, and peripheral vascular disease, that make them similarly high risk from a percutaneous standpoint. The complexity of LM PCI is dictated by the anatomy of the lesion. Stenosis could be limited to the ostium of the coronary artery, the body of the LM, or the length of the LM, and could involve the bifurcation with or without extension into the left anterior descending (LAD) or left circumflex coronary (LCX) arteries. Ostial or body obstructions in a long LM vessel are more desirable for PCI and stenting than bifurcation or trifurcation lesions.

Adequate planning and preparation is very important when tackling the LM anatomy. An appropriate strategy from the outset saves time and minimizes complications. Thrombotic complications during LM PCI are catastrophic, and thus pharmacotherapy in these cases should be thought through. Recent advances in pharmacotherapy have provided us with different regimens that achieve low thrombotic complications. Pretreatment with clopidogrel or prasugrel would be advisable, with sufficient time to achieve maximum platelet inhibition. Selected high-risk patients (Table 7h.1) may not tolerate ischemia as well and may benefit from prophylactic insertion of intra-aortic balloon pump (IABP), TandemHeart (CardiacAssist, Pittsburgh, PA), or an Impella device (Abiomed, Danvers, MA). If inserting one is not desirable, then at least securing access in the contralateral femoral artery before starting, in case one is needed, is recommended.

The choice of guide catheter is another critical step in planning the procedure and is dictated by the anatomy of the lesion. Coaxial alignment is an absolute requirement to allow ideal visualization, avoid complications, and minimize ischemia. Depending on the lesion location a 6 Fr guide would be reasonable choice for an ostial and midshaft lesion or a distal lesion with a small insignificant circumflex, unless rotablation is planned. However, if the lesion is at the bifurcation then an 8 Fr guide is needed to allow for kissing balloons at the end of the procedure. A left Judkins (JL) or similar guide would be preferable if 8 Fr system is used and avoids the need for an extra backup support or Amplatz guide, with deep engagement for an ostial and midshaft lesion. This allows guide adjustment for optimal stent positioning across the ostium before deployment.

If the lesion is ostial or mid shaft, then a single wire inserted into the LAD is adequate; however, if there is concern that plaque shift may occur in either branch, then double wire the LAD and CCA. The daily workhorse wire of choice is recommended in the majority of cases. If a hydrophilic-coated wire is used to cross the lesion, then it would be advisable to exchange it for a moderate support wire. Aggressive lesion preparation is the next step after securing the wires, and primary stenting must be avoided. Always predilate with an adequately sized balloon (avoid undersizing) to ensure satisfactory stent expansion. Although noncompliant balloons allow high-pressure inflations and better lesion preparation, they occasionally present difficulties when crossing the lesion. Balloon inflations should be brief and quick to shorten global ischemic time; inflation, however, should be repeated until a satisfactory result is

Table 7h.1 Indications for hemodynamic support for left main percutaneous coronary intervention

Consider hemodynamic support if:
1. Poor LV function
2. Systolic BP <100 mm Hg
3. RCA occlusion
4. Bifurcation location with calcifications
5. Concomitant complex distal disease
6. If in doubt

LV, left ventricular; BP, blood pressure; RCA, right coronary artery.

obtained. When faced with a calcified lesion, even if less than severe, consider rotational atherectomy (RA) as first step prior to balloon dilations, especially with ostial lesions.

The stenting technique depends on the location and branch involvement. Ostial lesions are occasionally rigid, with high recoil force. Thus, when stenting these lesions, the stent is positioned extending 1–2 mm into the aorta to provide adequate radial support (Fig. 7h.1). To succeed in this task, always check in multiple views, such as the right anterior oblique (RAO) cranial and left anterior oblique (LAO) caudal. Routinely perform a high-pressure postdilatation using a noncompliant balloon to flare the stent into the aorta. If the lesion extends distally into the bifurcation, then it becomes more complex and challenging. (The different classifications of bifurcation lesions and stenting techniques are discussed in detail in Chapter 7f.) Major side-branch occlusion during LM bifurcation PCI might cause disastrous clinical events; thus, it is vital to keep all branches open (Fig. 7h.2). It is important to wire the LM into the LAD as a first step to secure the vessel since it supplies approximately half of the myocardium. The need to wire and protect the circumflex artery is dictated by its size and the territory it supplies (Fig. 7h.3). Even if the intention is not to stent into the circumflex, it is better to protect it with a wire. As a rule of thumb, a single stent is always the better approach, producing a better long-term outcome when compared to double-stenting of the bifurcation.[2] If the circumflex ostium is free of disease, then provisional stenting is a reasonable approach; otherwise, choose

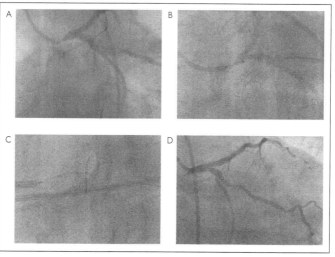

Figure 7h.1 Ostial stenosis. (A) Ostial left main stenosis. (B) A short stent is advanced across the ostium in an right anterior oblique (RAO) caudal view. (C) Postdilation is performed with a short balloon with high-pressure inflations. (D) Final angiographic result reveals adequate stent dilation.

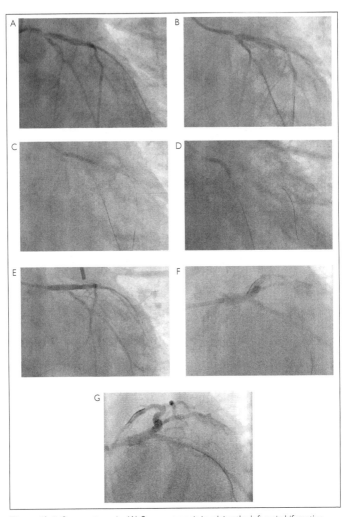

Figure 7h.2 Severe stenosis. (A) Severe stenosis involving the left main bifurcation. (B) Wiring of both the left anterior descending (LAD) and circumflex arteries was done. (C) Predilation of the LAD was performed. (D) Predilation of the circumflex ostium. (E) Stent deployed across the left main bifurcation into the LAD with a single-stent approach after pulling out the circumflex wire. (F) Rewiring of the circumflex artery and dilation of the side branch was performed, followed by kissing balloon angioplasty. (G) Final result reveals adequate stent dilation with <50% residual stenosis across the circumflex ostium.

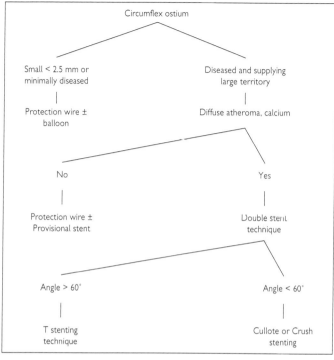

Figure 7h.3 Stepwise approach for the management of left main bifurcation stenosis determined by the circumflex artery disease and involvement.

a bifurcation stenting strategy according to the angle of the bifurcation. Always finish with simultaneous kissing balloons after any bifurcation stenting technique, as this is associated with lower restenosis and stent thrombosis rates. In choosing to use a bare metal stent (BMS) versus a DES, the LM is no different from the rest of the coronary tree. The long-term outcome is in favor of DES, with restenosis rates approaching the lower single digits for ostial stenting.[3] The bifurcation anatomy similarly carries a lower rate of restenosis, albeit higher rate of stent thrombosis[4]; however, this depends on the specific technique.

Intravascular ultrasound (IVUS) provides unique quantitative and qualitative information that is very helpful in LM PCI. Preintervention IVUS assesses lesion morphology and may guide treatment strategy, especially in deciding the use of RA. IVUS allows precise sizing of the LM, as compared to angiography, thus better balloon and stent size choice. Postintervention IVUS will more frequently reveal the need for additional balloon dilation and may help in optimally

Table 7h.2 **SYNTAX score and left main percutaneous coronary intervention outcomes**

	SYNTAX Score ≤ 34			SYNTAX Score >34		
	PCI (n = 257)	**CABG** (n = 273)	**P Value**	**PCI** (n = 85)	**CABG** (n = 204)	**P Value**
Mortality	8.1%	6.2%	NS	37.2%	8.5%	<0.001

The Synergy Between Percutaneous Coronary Intervention with TAXUS and Cardiac Surgery (SYNTAX) Score is a unique tool to score complexity of coronary artery disease. The score is calculated by a computer program consisting of sequential and interactive self-guided questions. The algorithm consists of 12 main questions. They can be divided in two groups: The first three determine the dominance, the total number of lesions, and the vessel segments involved per lesion, and they appear once. The maximum number of lesions allowed is 12, and each lesion is characterized by a number, 1–12. Each lesion can involve one or more segments. In this case, each vessel segment involved contributes to the lesion scoring. There is no limit to the number of segments involved per lesion. The last nine questions refer to adverse lesion characteristics and are repeated for each lesion.

expanding the stent. IVUS-guided LM stenting, especially with the use of a DES, may reduce mortality as compared to conventional angiography-guided PCI.[5]

Surveillance angiography is advocated following LM PCI to assess stent patency. This is driven by the fact that some of these patients' restenosis will manifest as sudden cardiac death. There is no consensus on when such angiography should be done, but most authorities support follow-up at 3–9 months, depending on whether a BMS or DES was used. With the widespread use of DESs in LM PCI, the circumflex ostium has been the most common site for restenosis, but the interventionist must be aware of pseudostenosis. It is always better to assess these lesions with fractional flow reserve (FFR) or IVUS prior to any further intervention. If there is restenosis involving one ostium, it can be managed with balloon angioplasty alone and follow-up.

Conclusion

Left main PCI is a high-risk interventional procedure that should be attempted by experienced interventional cardiologists only. While the data support a low rate of acute complications and better long-term outcomes, the stakes are high and complications are catastrophic. The Synergy Between PCI with TAXUS and Cardiac Surgery (SYNTAX) trial recently randomized patients with three-vessel and LM disease to either PCI or bypass surgery. Patients with LM disease and a low SYNTAX score had a favorable outcome as compared to those with a high score (Table 7h.2).[6] As we continue to refine the interventional equipment, with dedicated bifurcation stents and newer-generation DESs achieving low rates of restenosis and lower risk of late and very late stent thrombosis, the LM will become more appealing for percutaneous revascularization.

Practical Pearls

- Distal LM disease is technically more challenging than ostial or shaft disease.
- Circulatory support is not routinely recommended, but it should be considered in high-risk patients.
- A single-stent technique is preferable, with lower restenosis rates.
- IVUS is useful in assessing vessel size and final stenting result.
- Always finish with simultaneous kissing balloons after a bifurcation stenting.

References

1. Tan WA, Tamai H, Park SJ, et al. Long-term clinical outcomes after unprotected left main trunk percutaneous revascularization in 279 patients. *Circulation.* 2001;104(14):1609-1614.

2. Palmerini T, Sangiorgi D, Marzocchi A, et al. Ostial and midshaft lesions vs. bifurcation lesions in 1111 patients with unprotected left main coronary artery stenosis treated with drug-eluting stents: results of the survey from the Italian Society of Invasive Cardiology. *Eur Heart J.* 2009:ehp223.

3. Chieffo A, Park SJ, Valgimigli M, et al. Favorable long-term outcome after drug-eluting stent implantation in nonbifurcation lesions that involve unprotected left main coronary artery: a multicenter registry. *Circulation.* 2007;116(2):158-162.

4. Chieffo A, Park S-J, Meliga E, et al. Late and very late stent thrombosis following drug-eluting stent implantation in unprotected left main coronary artery: a multi-centre registry. *Eur Heart J.* 2008;29(17):2108-2115.

5. Park S-J, Kim Y-H, Park D-W, et al. Impact of intravascular ultrasound guidance on long-term mortality in stenting for unprotected left main coronary artery stenosis. *Circ Cardiovasc Intervent.* 2009;2(3):167-177.

6. Capodanno D, Di Salvo ME, Cincotta G, Miano M, Tamburino C, Tamburino C. Usefulness of the SYNTAX score for predicting clinical outcome after percutaneous coronary intervention of unprotected left main coronary artery disease. *Circ Cardiovasc Intervent.* 2009;2(4):302-308.

Chapter 8

Embolic Protection Devices, Rotational Atherectomy, Mechanical Thrombectomy Devices, and More

Ion S. Jovin, Allyne Topaz, Pritam R. Polkampally, and On Topaz

The armamentarium of the interventional cardiologist should include classical tools such as balloon catheters and stents, as well as several special devices. Such devices include embolic protection systems, rotational atherectomy (RA) devices, and mechanical thrombectomy devices.

Embolic Protection Systems

Embolization of the microvasculature leads to the phenomenon of slow reflow or no reflow.[1] Embolic protection devices (EPDs) are used to prevent the propagation of thrombus or atheromatous material downstream from percutaneous coronary intervention (PCI) sites. Embolic protection devices are currently used in the treatment of saphenous vein graft lesions.

The EPDs can be classified into three broad categories: filter-based, and proximal and distal flow-occlusion devices. The proximal and distal occlusion devices occlude the flow and usually involve some type of aspiration. Examples of the filter-based devices include the FilterWire-EZ (Boston Scientific, Natick, MA) (Fig. 8.1a–c), the SpideRX protection device (eV3), and the Rubicon system (Rubicon Medical, Salt Lake City, UT). The Proxis embolic protection system (St. Jude Medical, St. Paul, MN) is a proximal occlusion device. Distal occlusion devices include the PercuSurge GuardWire (Medtronic Vascular, Danvers, MA) and the TriActive system (Kensey Nash, Exton, PA). These systems retrieve smaller particles but share some limitations with the distal filter devices. The characteristics of EPDs are presented in Table 8.1.

Patient Preparation

The use of EPDs does not require any special patient preparation, other than the standard anticoagulation therapy for percutaneous intervention. Most of

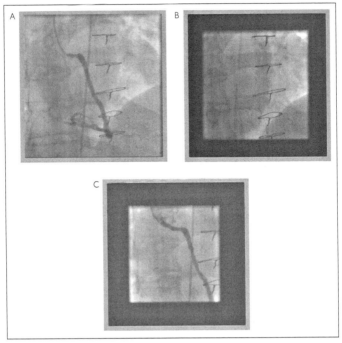

Figure 8.1 Use of EZ FilterWire distal protection device in a patient with significant chest pain and inferior ischemia on stress echo. (A) Ostial lesion in a saphenous vein graft to the right posterior descending artery. (B) EZ FilterWire in mid section of the target vessel. (C) Final results demonstrating no residual stenosis after stent placement. The patient remained asymptomatic, and a repeat myocardial perfusion stress test 9 months post intervention showed no evidence of ischemia.

these devices are userfriendly, as they were initially designed for urgent situations such as primary angioplasty for acute myocardial infarction (MI).

Technique

Most EPDs (except for the Proxis; see below) are inserted over the guidewire.

The FilterWire is a prototypical example of a commonly used EPD. Listed here are step-by-step instructions for its use.

1. Under fluoroscopic imaging, steer the FilterWire System into the target vessel. Using a two-handed technique, torque the protection wire with one hand and advance the EZ Delivery Sheath with the other hand.
2. Advance the FilterWire System across the lesion until the apex of the filter loop can be deployed in the recommended minimum landing zone (≥2.5 cm for FilterWire EZ System 2.25–3.5 mm; and ≥3.0 cm for FilterWire EZ System 3.5–5.5 mm).

Table 8.1 General features and examples of embolic protection devices

Filter-based Devices	Proximal Occlusion Devices	Distal Occlusion Devices
Pros: Antegrade flow preserved	Pros: Lesion crossing protected	Pros: Protection independent of particle size
Optimal visualization	Cons: Flow obstruction may cause ischemia	Cons: Lesion crossing not protected
Cons: Lesion crossing not protected		Flow obstruction may cause ischemia
FilterWire EZ	Proxis	GuardWire
6 Fr guide compatible	7 Fr guide compatible	7 Fr guide compatible
3.2 Fr crossing profile	Balloon occlusion of proximal vessel	Balloon occlusion of distal vessel
Own guidewire	Aspiration of thromboembolic material	Aspiration of thromboembolic material through separate catheter
Basket diameter 3.5–5 mm		
110 µm pores		
SpideRX		TriActive sytem
6 Fr guide compatible		7 Fr guide compatible
Own guidewire		Balloon occlusion of distal vessel
Basket size 3–7 mm		Aspiration of thromboembolic material through guide catheter
110 µm pores		
Rubicon		
6 Fr guide compatible		
2 Fr crossing profile		
Own guidewire		
100 µm pores		

3. Once the protection wire is advanced past the lesion, slide the wire torquer along the protection wire and secure it against the hemostasis valve.

4. Deploy the filter by holding the protection wire in place with the wire torquer pressed against the hemostasis valve while simultaneously retracting the EZ Delivery Sheath.

5. Inject contrast media to verify that the filter is in the proper position and that there is adequate flow.

6. After completion of the procedure, and while maintaining wire position distal to the lesion, advance the EZ Retrieval Sheath over the wire past any deployed stent(s) until the tip of the EZ Retrieval Sheath reaches the protection wire's catheter stop.

7. Gently and slowly retract the protection wire and filter loop back into the EZ Retrieval Sheath until resistance is felt.

8. Remove the FilterWire EZ System from the patient, ensuring that the hemostasis valve is fully opened prior to FilterWire EZ System removal.

Proxis Device

The Proxis device requires a slightly different approach:

1. The recommended technique[2] is to insert the Proxis catheter into the guide catheter.

2. A guidewire of choice is inserted into the catheter's hemostatic valve, advanced through the Proxis catheter, and positioned just proximal to the target lesion.

3. The operator then preloads the desired interventional device on the guide-wire and advances through the Proxis catheter toward the distal end of the protection catheter.

4. Next, the sealing balloon should be inflated. The lesion is crossed with the guidewire. While maintaining suspended antegrade blood flow, the inter-ventional device is advanced onto the lesion, activated, then removed from the vessel.

5. The suspended fluid and debris from the vessel are gently aspirated with the aspiration syringe. Then the deflate button is pressed, and the one-way stopcock is opened to the inflation device in order to deflate the Proxis sealing balloon. Aspiration is continued until a total of 20 cc of fluid has been removed.

6. The target vessel is reassessed angiographically. Upon completion of the intervention, the Proxis catheter and the guide catheter are removed as a single unit.

Results

Selected trials comparing the use of EPDs to standard angioplasty (without protection device) are summarized in Table 8.2.The EPDs are useful adjuncts, especially in percutaneous interventions in saphenous vein graft lesions,[3] and have been shown to be efficacious in reducing the rate of periprocedural infarc-tion.[4] The EPDs do not seem to improve outcomes when used in the setting of acute ST elevation MI, but have a Class I indication for saphenous vein graft interventions. There does not appear to be a significant difference between the FilterWire device and the AngioGuard device[5] in terms of death, MI, or target vessel revascularization at 30 days.

In peripheral endovascular interventions, EPDs such as the AngioGuard, FilterWire, Accunet, and SpideRX are also utilized successfully, although their main utilization is in carotid interventions. The application of these devices in renal and lower extremity interventions is limited.[1]

Rotational Atherectomy Devices

Rotational atherectomy (Rotablator, Boston Scientific, Natick, MA) was intro-duced in the mid 1980s, initially as a peripheral plaque debulking technology,[5,6] followed by coronary applications. Rotational atherectomy is based upon the principle of "differential cutting" (Fig. 8.2).[6] The aim of the device is to

Table 8.2 Trials comparing embolic protection devices with percutaneous coronary intervention without protection

Trial	Device	Patients (n)	Setting	Main Endpoint	Outcome
SAFER (Baim DS et al. *Circulation*. 2002;105:1285)	GuardWire	801	Saphenous vein graft intervention	30-day MACE	GuardWire improved outcomes
EMERALD (Stone GW et al. *JAMA*. 2005;293:1063)	GuardWire	501	Primary percutaneous coronary intervention	ST segment resolution and infarct size	No difference
PROMISE (Gick et al. *Circulation*. 2005;112:1062)	Filterwire EZ	200	Primary percutaneous coronary intervention in STEMI and NSTEMI	Flow velocity in infarct related artery	No difference

MACE, major adverse cardiac events; NSTEMI, non-ST elevation myocardial infarction; STEMI, ST elevation myocardial infarction.

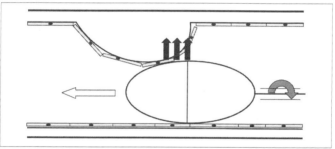

Figure 8.2 Principles of rotational atherectomy ("differential cutting"). The rotablator burr advances forward (*white arrow*) along the atherosclerotic vessel, rotating at 160,000 rpm (*gray arrow*). Note that the leading half, which is coated with diamond chips, interacts (*black arrows*) with the hardened, calcified plaque (*top*) and not with the normal, elastic vessel wall (*bottom*).

exclusively remove hard, calcified lesions by the action of a diamond-coated burr rotating at high speed. The normal elastic tissue is not affected by the rotating burr. This technology was expected to improve plaque removal and thereby reduce restenosis rate when compared to balloon angioplasty.[7] Currently, RA is used mainly in calcified lesions for facilitation of stent deployment.[8] Rotational atherectomy should be avoided in tortuous vessels, as excessive vessel tortuosity and angulation is significantly associated with perforation, as demonstrated in large case series and randomized trials.

Patient Preparation

Standard anticoagulation should be employed. When atherectomy of a proximal lesion in a dominant right coronary artery is planned, prophylactic placement of a temporary pacemaker wire in the right ventricle is recommended because of the concern for high-degree arteriovenous (AV) block. Some interventionalists advocate the use of intravenous aminophylline (500 mg in a short infusion at the beginning of the procedure) to prevent AV block and to avoid the need for a temporary pacemaker.

Technique

1. The 325-cm, 0.009-inch rotablation wires vary in degree of stiffness, ranging from floppy to extra support. The tip is composed of a 0.014-inch radiopaque coil. The rotablator is backloaded on the guidewire. Available burr sizes (in mm) are: 1.25, 1.5, 1.75, 2.0, 2.15, 2.25, and 2.50. The smallest two sizes can be accommodated by a large-lumen 6 Fr guide catheter; higher sized catheters are needed for the larger burrs. As a rule, the burr-to-artery diameter ratio should be 0.7 or smaller. The burr rotates at 140,000–160,000 rpm, and the drive shaft is encased by a Teflon sheath through which a heparinized flush solution containing a proprietary lubricant emulsion (Rotaglide) is pumped.

2. The rotablation is performed while advancing the burr across the calcified lesion. Most operators recommend ablation using a "pecking" motion, in which brief periods of debulking alternate with burr retraction. Forceful advancement of the burr should be avoided as it causes decelerations (>5,000 rpm); such decelerations are associated with excessive heat

Table 8.3 Selected trials evaluating the use of rotational atherectomy

Trial	Comparison with	Patients (n)	Setting	Main Endpoint	Outcome
COBRA (Dill T et al. Eur Heart J. 2000;21:1727)	Balloon angioplasty	502	Complex lesions	6-month restenosis and MACE	No difference
DART (Mauri L et al. Am Heart J. 2003;145;847)	Balloon angioplasty	446	Vessels <3 mm	12-month target vessel failure	No difference
ARTIST (vom Dahl J et al. Circulation. 2002:105:583)	Balloon angioplasty	298	In-stent restenosis	6-month restenosis and MACE	Angioplasty better
ROSTER (Sharma S et al. Am Heart J. 2004;147:16)	Balloon angioplasty	200	In-stent restenosis	9-month target lesion revascularization	Rotablation better

MACE, major adverse cardiac events.

generation and resultant vascular trauma. If the burr detaches, it can be retrieved by removal of the guidewire.

3. Final removal of the burr upon completion of the rotablation is set with the console on "Dynaglide" mode.

Several trials comparing RA with other techniques are presented in Table 8.3.

Results

Rotablation is a useful tool for calcified lesions that cannot be dilated by standard balloon angioplasty. As a stand-alone technique, rotablation is not superior to bare metal stenting. Trials comparing rotablation with drug-eluting stenting are not available. This atherectomy technique is also used successfully in peripheral vascular interventions, when the primary goal is debulking.[8] Several other types of atherectomy devices are also used in peripheral interventions. These devices include directional atherectomy (SilverHawk, eV3, Plymouth, MN), orbital atherectomy (CSI DiamondBack 360), and RA devices (Pathway JetStream; Pathway Medical Technologies, Inc., Redmond, WA).

Thrombectomy Devices

Thrombectomy devices are used in the treatment of thrombus-containing lesions. Their target is to eliminate distal embolization and the occurrence of no-reflow.[9] This section delineates mechanical aspiration catheters, the rheolytic atherectomy (AngioJet) catheter, and the excimer laser.

Aspiration Thrombectomy Catheters

Aspiration catheters consist of mechanical and suction devices. Manual aspiration systems include the DiverCE (Invatec, Roncadelle, Italy), Export (Medtronic, Minneapolis, MN), QuickCat (Kensey Nash, Exton, PA), and Pronto (Vascular Solutions, Minneapolis, MN) catheters.

Manual aspiration catheters are valuable because they are quick and easy to use, as well as relatively inexpensive. Recent meta-analyses indicate that aspiration thrombectomy is associated with improved survival, as well as decreased angiographic evidence of distal embolization ST elevation MI (STEMI).[10–14]

Technique for Aspiration Thrombectomy

1. Advance a standard coronary wire distal to the culprit lesion.
2. Advance the aspiration thrombectomy catheter over the coronary wire to the culprit lesion.
3. Activate aspiration by opening suction syringe to patient.
4. While suction is occurring, make several gentle passes along the culprit lesion.
5. Remove the device when the suction syringe is full of blood.

AngioJet

Specific thrombectomy devices include the AngioJet rheolytic thrombectomy system (Possis Medical Inc., Minneapolis, MN), which uses the Bernoulli effect, created by a saline jet, to remove debris. The phenomenon involves thrombus aspiration and microscopic fragmentation.

Patient preparation incorporates a standard anticoagulation regimen.

After priming of the console, the catheter is connected to the attached tubing; 4 and 5 Fr AngioJet catheters are available in both over-the-wire and rapid-exchange formats. The largest catheters (XVG and AVX) are used for large saphenous vein grafts or for peripheral thrombotic vessels. The AngioJet catheter is activated in a slow advancement mode along the entire length of the target thrombus in an antegrade and retrograde fashion. It can be combined with direct pharmacolytic therapy in activation mode using the "pulsed spray technique."[15]

The AngioJet is most successful in removing fresh thrombus, but it can also be useful in organized thrombus. In the presence of a large thrombus burden or resistant clot, the administration of lytics selectively into the target vessel in conjunction with the AngioJet has been studied.[16,17] Clinical studies have shown that the AngioJet does not cause significant vessel damage. Several trials, such as VEGAS 1, VEGAS 2, and AIMI,[18,19] have studied the usefulness of the AngioJet catheter in the treatment of thrombus-laden lesions and in the setting of primary angioplasty.

Results

Aspiration thrombectomy catheters are simple and useful devices for primary PCI, and they are associated with improved survival. The AngioJet is an effective tool for treatment of thrombus-laden lesions in native coronary arteries and saphenous vein grafts in the context of acute MI, and acute coronary and ischemic peripheral syndromes. Recently, it has been introduced for treatment of pulmonary embolism.[20] The current evidence does not support the routine use of the AngioJet system in primary PCI. The ongoing JETSTENT (AngioJET thrombectomy and STENTing for treatment of acute MI) trial will provide much needed information on the role of rheolytic thrombectomy as an adjunct to primary PCI.

Excimer Laser

The ultraviolet 308 nm excimer laser (CVX-300, Spectranetics, Colorado Springs, CO) has the unique abilities of concomitant plaque and thrombus vaporization. It safely ablates underlying atherosclerotic plaque and facilitates subsequent stent placement. This device promotes rapid thrombus clearance and suppresses platelet aggregation.[21] The excimer laser is currently used for treatment of thrombus-laden lesions in saphenous vein grafts (Fig. 8.3a–d) and native coronary arteries in acute MI and unstable angina.[22] It is a useful tool for the debulking of in-stent restenosis, ostial lesions, and chronic total occlusions.[23]

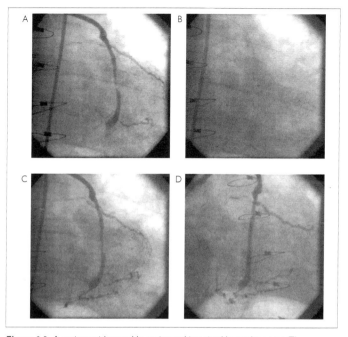

Figure 8.3 A patient with unstable angina and impaired hemodynamics. The target lesion is the saphenous vein graft to the distal obtuse marginal (OM) artery. (A) Preintervention view demonstrating 99% eccentric thrombotic lesion in the mid saphenous vein graft. The graft is occluded distally by a large thrombus. (B) A 1.7 mm concentric excimer laser catheter at the target lesion. (C) Post laser debulking of the underlying plaque and associated thrombus. (D) Final angiogram following adjunct stenting demonstrating patency of the target lesion and the distal segment of the graft. The patient improved clinically.

Patient Preparation

Routine patient preparation and anticoagulation for percutaneous intervention are required.

Technique

1. The latest laser catheters have improved fiber array with concentric or eccentric tip configuration. The rapid-exchange concentric coronary catheters are available in 0.9 mm, 1.4 mm, 1.7 mm, and 2.0 mm sizes. Eccentric catheters are available in 1.7 mm and 2.0 mm sizes. The eccentric catheters are reserved for circumferential debulking in in-stent stenosis lesions for markedly eccentric lesions.

2. Proper lasing technique is crucial to the success of laser angioplasty.[24] Because iodinated contrast has a significant potentiating effect on peak pressure waves, removal of contrast before lasing is mandatory to avoid vessel trauma. This is done by injecting saline into the guide catheter.

3. Slow advancement (0.5 mm/sec) of the laser catheter during activation is recommended. The computer lasing program within the laser console limits each lasing train to 5 seconds, except for 10 seconds with the X-80 0.9-mm catheter.

4. The patient and the catheterization laboratory staff should wear special protective goggles.

Results

Laser angioplasty has been studied in acute coronary and peripheral ischemic syndromes for thrombus-laden lesions, in-stent restenosis, and chronic total occlusions.

Conclusion

Embolic protection, RA, and aspiration thrombectomy tools are used in acute coronary and peripheral ischemic syndromes. This includes interventions in native coronary vessels; saphenous vein grafts; calcified, nondilatable lesions; and chronic total occlusions. In the era of drug-eluting stents, these devices are frequently used as part of a prestenting strategy.

Practical Pearls

• The catheterization laboratory staff should be familiar with preparation of the relevant niche devices. Frequent in-service training is recommended.

• When performing interventions on saphenous veins, use filter-based protection devices to reduce the potential for distal embolization or no-reflow phenomenon.

• Ensure adequate guiding catheter and guidewire support. This is important when using a 6 Fr EBU, XB, or Amplatz left guiding catheter configuration. An Amplatz left guide catheter is useful for technically demanding left coronary interventions. For intervention in an anatomically challenging right coronary artery, both Amplatz right or Amplatz left shapes can provide adequate support.

• In challenging lesions, first cross the target with a soft-tip, flexible guidewire. Then exchange it for a stiff, supportive guidewire. This will significantly enhance subsequent device delivery and improve its utilization.

References

1. Roffi M, Mukherjee D. Current role of emboli protection devices in percutaneous coronary and vascular interventions. *Am Heart J.* 2009;157(2):263-270.

2. http://www.sjm.com/_MediaAssets/documents/resources/IFU_Proxis_System_CAN.pdf

3. Bates ER. Aspirating and filtering atherothrombotic debris during percutaneous coronary intervention. *JACC Cardiovasc Interv.* 2008;1(3):265-267.

4. Baim DS, Wahr D, George B, et al. Randomized trial of a distal embolic protection device during percutaneous intervention of saphenous vein aorto-coronary bypass grafts. *Circulation.* 2002;105(11):1285-1290.

5. Ahn SS, Auth D, Marcus DR, Moore WS. Removal of focal atheromatous lesions by angioscopically guided high-speed rotary atherectomy. Preliminary experimental observations. *J Vasc Surg.* 1988;7(2):292-300.

6. Hansen DD, Auth DC, Vracko R, Ritchie JL. Rotational atherectomy in atherosclerotic rabbit iliac arteries. *Am Heart J.* 1988;115(1 Pt 1):160-165.

7. Tran T, Brown M, Lasala J. An evidence-based approach to the use of rotational and directional coronary atherectomy in the era of drug-eluting stents: when does it make sense? *Catheter Cardiovasc Interv.* 2008;72(5):650-662.

8. Shrikhande GV, McKinsey JF. Use and abuse of atherectomy: where should it be used? *Semin Vasc Surg.* 2008;21(4):204-209.

9. Kelly RV, Cohen MG, Stoutter GA. Mechanical thrombectomy options in complex percutaneous coronary interventions. *Catheter Cardiovasc Interv.* 2006;68(6):917-928.

10. Burzotta F, Testa L, Giannico F, et al. Adjunctive devices in primary or rescue PCI: A meta-analysis of randomized trials. *Int J Cardiol.* 2008;123:313-321

11. De Luca G, Suryapranata H, Stone GW, Antoniucci D, Neumann FJ, Chiariello M. Adjunctive mechanical devices to prevent distal embolization in patients undergoing mechanical revascularization for acute myocardial infarction: a meta-analysis of randomized trials. *Am Heart J.* 2007;153:343-353.

12. Svilaas T, Vlaar PJ, van der Horst IC, et al. Thrombus aspiration during primary percutaneous coronary intervention. *N Engl J Med.* 2008;358(6):557-567.

13. Burzotta F, Trani C, Romagnoli E, et al. Manual thrombus-aspiration improves myocardial reperfusion: the randomized evaluation of the effect of mechanical reduction of distal embolization by thrombus-aspiration in primary and rescue angioplasty (REMEDIA) trial. *J Am Coll Cardiol.* 2005;46(2):371-376.

14. Bavry AA, Kumbhani DJ, Bhatt DL. Role of adjunctive thrombectomy and embolic protection devices in acute myocardial infarction: a comprehensive meta-analysis of randomized trials. *Eur Heart J.* 2008;29:2989-3001.

15. Allie DE, Hebert CJ, Lirtzman MD, et al. Novel simultaneous combination chemical thrombolysis/rheolytic thrombectomy therapy for acute critical limb ischemia: the power-pulse spray technique. *Catheter Cardiovasc Interv.* 2004;63(4):512-522.

16. Topaz O. Editorial. On the hostile massive thrombus and the means to eradicate it. *Cath Cardiovasc Intervent.* 2005;65:280-281.

17. Topaz O. Editorial. Revascularization of thrombus laden lesions in AMI: the burden on the interventionalist. *J Invas Cardiol.* 2007;19:324-325

18. Kuntz RE, Baim DS, Cohen DJ, et al. A trial comparing rheolytic thrombectomy with intracoronary urokinase for coronary and vein graft thrombus (the Vein Graft AngioJet Study [VeGAS 2]). *Am J Cardiol.* 2002;89(3):326-330.

19. Ali A, Cox D, Dib N, et al. Rheolytic thrombectomy with percutaneous coronary intervention for infarct size reduction in acute myocardial infarction: 30-day results from a multicenter randomized study. *J Am Coll Cardiol.* 2006;48(2):244-252.

20. Margheri M. Early and long-term clinical results of AngioJet rheolytic thrombectomy in patients with acute pulmonary embolism. *Am J Cardiol.* 2009;101:252-258.

21. Topaz O, Minisi AJ, Bernardo NL, et al. Alteration of platelet aggregation kinetics with ultraviolet laser emission: the stunned platelet phenomenon. *Thromb Haemost.* 2001;86:1087-1093.

22. Topaz O, Ebersole D, Das T, et al. Excimer laser angioplasty in acute myocardial infarction (the CARMEL multicenter trial). *Am J Cardiol.* 2004;93(6):694-701.

23. Topaz O. Lasers in CTO. In: Waksman R, Saito S, eds. *Chronic total occlusions.* Chichester, UK: Wiley, 2009; 150-164.

24. Topaz O. Laser. In: Topol EJ, ed., *Textbook of interventional cardiology*, 4th ed. Philadelphia: WB Saunders, 2003; 675-703.

Chapter 9

Complications of Percutaneous Coronary Intervention: Stent Loss and Retrieval, Perforation, Access Site Hematoma, Arteriovenous Fistula, Radial Artery Access

Sharat Koul

This chapter reviews a set of complications related to percutaneous coronary intervention (PCI) and provides practical insights on how to troubleshoot and manage them.

Stent Loss

Stents are used in the majority of PCI because they improve angiographic outcomes and reduce the need for repeat revascularization.[1] With prepackaged balloon-mounted stents, stent loss is rare, but it can be a serious complication, resulting in either coronary and/or systemic embolization.

In a retrospective series of over 11,000 interventions, stent loss occurred in 0.32% of the procedures. Predictors for stent loss were lesion calcification and significant proximal angulation.[2] Stent loss led to an increased need for emergency coronary artery bypass graft surgery (5% vs 0.4%; p <0.001) and higher incidence of bleeding requiring transfusion (24% vs 7%; p <0.001).[2]

Management

There are a few described techniques to recover stents. The first consideration when deciding on the appropriate method is whether the stent is still on the percutaneous transluminal coronary angioplasty (PTCA) wire.

The most common situation seen with stent loss occurs when the stent gets stripped but remains on the PTCA wire. In this event, the following two approaches should be considered. The easiest one is the small-balloon technique (Fig. 9.1).[3] The other technique is called the two-wire technique (Fig. 9.2).[4]

If the stent is not on the wire, a loop snare can be used to retrieve the stent (Fig. 9.3).[5] Loop snares are available commercially (Amplatz Goose Neck Snare;

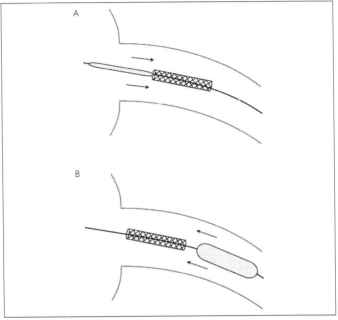

Figure 9.1 Small balloon technique. A small percutaneous transluminal coronary angioplasty (PTCA) balloon is advanced over the wire (A) and through the stent. The balloon is inflated distal to the stent (B) and withdrawn along with the stent into the guide catheter.

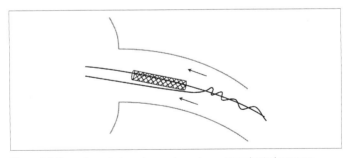

Figure 9.2 Two-wire technique. A second percutaneous transluminal coronary angioplasty (PTCA) wire is advanced distal to the stent, and both guidewires are twisted several times to cause entanglement of the distal tips, then both wires are removed along with the lost stent.

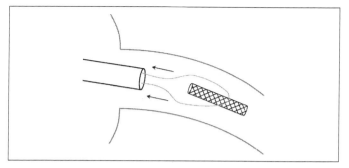

Figure 9.3 Snare retrieval. Recovering the stent requires advancing a loop over the stent then retracting the wire to trap the stent between the wire and guide catheter. Complete recovery with externalization of the stent is accomplished by applying continuous traction to the wire to prevent loss of the stent while removing the guide.

eV3, Plymouth, MN), or one can be prepared using a guide catheter and a long PTCA guidewire.

Special Issues

If the stent is lost in the peripheral vasculature, the aforementioned techniques can be used for recovery, but a few other tools are also available that can be useful. A lost stent can be retrieved using biliary forceps, the Cook retained-fragment retriever (Cook, Bloomington, IN), or a basket retrieval device.[6,7] These devices are larger in size and can only be used in larger vessels.

If the stent is not retrieved, the "crush" technique can be employed (see Fig. 9.4 and Table 9.1).

Practical Pearls

• Minimize stent loss with lesion preparation (PTCA/rotational atherectomy) before stenting.

• Avoid direct stenting in high-risk lesions (calcification, angulation).

• Ensure adequate anticoagulation during stent retrieval due to risk of thrombotic complications associated with longer procedural time and/or simultaneous use of more interventional equipment.

Arterial Perforation

Coronary perforation is a rare but dreaded complication of PCI. In a series of over 12,000 PCI procedures, perforation was observed in only 0.5% of cases. This complication was seen more often with devices intended to remove or ablate tissue (atherectomy, laser) and was more prevalent in the elderly and female populations. Oversizing of PTCA balloons has been shown to be associated with a greater risk of perforation.[8]

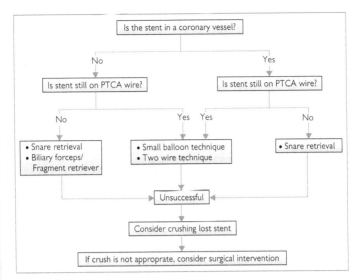

Figure 9.4 Algorithm for management of stent loss.

Table 9.1 Crush technique

- Deployment of an overlying stent, thereby "crushing" the lost stent
- Certain locations such as left main/left anterior descending artery may pose unacceptable risk.
- Increases risk of restenosis, which may be mitigated with use of drug-eluting stent
- Technique can be used in peripheral vascular system as well.

Ellis described the classification system for coronary perforations shown in Figure 9.5.[8] It is critical to understand these descriptions, because they assist in determining the optimal management.

Management

The algorithm for management of perforation is summarized in Figure 9.6.

For type 2 or 3 perforations, the use of polytetrafluoroethylene (PTFE)-covered stents is indicated, and the method of their delivery is described here (Fig. 9.7).[9]

Special Issues

The bulk of significant perforations are produced by tears in the arterial wall. Perforations due to hydrophilic PTCA wires tend to be benign since the defects produced are very small, pinpoint lesions. Although this type of perforation can be treated with techniques already described, other unique modalities also are described here.

If the perforation has occurred at the distal tips of the epicardial vessels, microcoil embolization can be performed.[10] With delivery of the coils to the

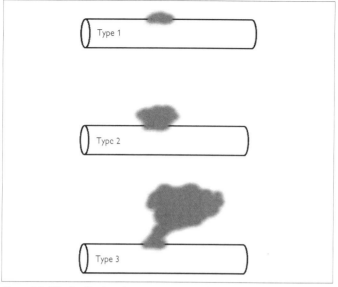

Figure 9.5 Ellis classification of coronary artery perforations. Type 1 (*top*) perforations are described as an extraluminal crater without extravasation of dye. These lesions are quite difficult to identify on angiography and are often mistaken for dissections. They rarely result in tamponade or any significant ischemia. Type 2 (*middle*) perforations produce myocardial or pericardial blush with frank contrast jet extravasation. These can be treated with prolonged balloon inflation, usually producing a reasonable angiographic result. Reversal of heparin with protamine is often not performed with this type of perforation. There is a possibility of developing late tamponade (up to 24 hours) with these patients, so that observation in a critical care setting may be appropriate. Type 3 (*bottom*) perforations produce a contrast jet with ≥1 mm diameter size opening and are associated with a high incidence of major adverse events (death, emergency coronary artery bypass graft surgery, tamponade). Prolonged balloon inflation is often not sufficient, and use of polytetrafluoroethylene (PTFE) covered stents may be the only means of avoiding emergency cardiac surgery. Cessation of all antiplatelet agents and reversal of heparin with protamine should also be performed emergently.

distal points in the vessel, the spot of injury can be plugged effectively. Another maneuver is to use a PTCA balloon catheter to deliver thrombin to the distal vessel, causing closure of the distal artery and the point of bleeding.[11]

Practical Pearls

- Keep a PTCA balloon readily available when performing higher-risk procedures (atherectomy), in case of perforation.
- Current PTFE-covered stents require 7 Fr guiding catheters for deployment.
- Despite the fact that most perforations can be handled percutaneously, it is our practice to contact surgical backup once perforation is identified, in case of a failed attempt.

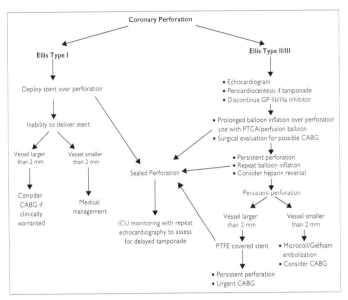

Figure 9.6 Algorithm for management of coronary perforation. Adapted from Rogers JH, Lasala JM. Coronary artery dissection and perforation complicating percutaneous coronary intervention. *J Invasive Cardiol.* 2004;16(9):493-499, with permission of the publisher.

Femoral Artery Hematoma

In PCI, the most common complication is bleeding related to arterial access. We shall discuss the specific complications of hematoma development and arteriovenous (AV) fistula formation in this section. The incidence of bleeding complication/hematoma formation is quite low in current practice (<1%).[12,13] Factors associated with bleeding are detailed in Table 9.2.

Management

The most common presentation of bleeding is an external groin hematoma. This can be managed with simple manual compression. If compression is unsuccessful, surgical cutdown under local anesthesia can be performed to acquire hemostasis. If the puncture site is below the inguinal ligament, an endovascular approach should be avoided because stent placement in this region is associated with multiple problems.[14]

Bleeding can also result in a retroperitoneal hematoma. Volume resuscitation is often adequate for this situation, but with refractory hypotension, an endovascular approach, described in Table 9.3, can be selectively attempted.

When an endovascular approach is not possible, these patients may need surgery to control the bleeding.

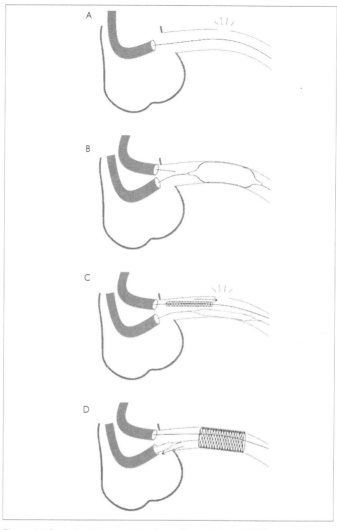

Figure 9.7 Steps for deployment of polytetrafluoroethylene (PTFE)-covered stent. (A) Perforation is seen with coronary angiography. (B) A second guiding catheter is placed in the ascending aorta. At this point, the usual situation is that the initial guide is engaged in the coronary ostium with an interventional wire and percutaneous transluminal coronary angioplasty (PTCA) balloon in place, occluding the point of perforation. With care, the first guide is slightly withdrawn to allow engagement of the coronary artery with the second guide. Through this guide is advanced an interventional wire. (C, D) In rapid succession, the PTCA balloon is deflated and withdrawn. The second interventional wire is then passed by the lesion and the PTFE-covered stent is quickly advanced and deployed.

Table 9.2 Risk factors for femoral artery bleeding complications

- Renal insufficiency
- Female gender
- High arterial puncture
- Use of glycoprotein IIb/IIIa inhibitors

Table 9.3 Endovascular approach to femoral arterial bleeding

- Clinical suspicion for femoral artery bleeding/retroperitoneal hemorrhage
- Access obtained in contralateral femoral artery
- Angiogram performed of iliofemoral system
- If perforation noted above inguinal ligament, a cross-over sheath is placed in the common iliac artery
- A covered stent (iCast balloon expandable stent, Atrium Medical, Hudson, NH) or a stent graft (Fluency, Bard Medical, Covington, GA) can be placed to obtain permanent hemostasis.

Femoral Arteriovenous Fistula

The overall incidence of AV fistula formation (Fig. 9.8) is also quite low (<1%). Risk factors for their development are shown in Table 9.4.

Arteriovenous fistula should be suspected in patients with a bruit present over the femoral artery after an intervention. These can be diagnosed by performing a vascular ultrasound examination.

Management

Management of this complication depends on the overall size of the fistula. If the fistula is small and does not involve the common femoral artery, an endovascular delivery of microcoils to close off the communication may be sufficient. If the fistula is larger, surgical ligation of the artery may be needed.[14] The AV fistula can be closed with a Perclose device (Abbot Vascular, Abbot Park, IL), but this technique is not standard of care and should be performed only by those with the required expertise.

Minimizing the risk of access bleeding complications is done with use of fluoroscopy to delineate anatomical landmarks and the use of SMART Needle technology (Escalon Vascular, New Berlin, WI) as needed. As expected, the judicious use of antithrombotics/antiplatelet agents reduces bleeding complications.

In regards to arterial closure devices (ACDs), there are little clear-cut, prospective data to either support or discourage their use.[15,16] Their use should be individualized, as assessed by the interventionalist in terms of benefits from earlier ambulation versus the associated risks.

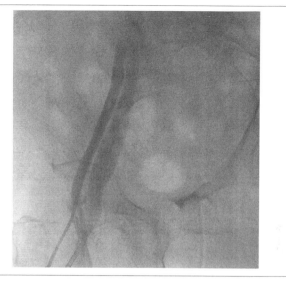

Figure 9.8 Femoral arteriovenous fistula.

Table 9.4 Risk factors for arteriovenous fistula formation

- High heparin dosage
- Coumadin therapy
- Puncture of the left groin
- Arterial hypertension
- Female gender

Practical Pearls

- Femoral access under active fluoroscopy to delineate vascular calcification can aid with arterial puncture.
- Micropuncture kit usage can minimize the risk of access complications.

Complications of Intervention via the Radial Artery

With the importance of periprocedural bleeding and prognosis with PCI,[17–19] radial arterial access is attractive since it seems to afford a lessened bleeding risk.[20] The superficial nature of the artery makes compressibility very simple. The occurrence of a hematoma and AV fistula formation is quite rare.[21]

The most common complication seen is radial arterial occlusion. The sequela of this tends not to be significant, with few problems reported in the literature.[21] In the event that this leads to hand ischemia, a typical approach is prompt heparinization of the patient, with a surgical evaluation for thrombus removal.

Arterial spasm is a common issue seen with radial arterial access. This is treated with the use of intra-arterial vasodilators. If spasm is not recognized, introduction of interventional wires and catheters can produce further injury, including perforation and dissection of the upper extremity arterial system. In addition, spasm can make removal of the arterial sheath difficult, and can result in avulsion of the radial artery. These complications are extremely rare with the use of contemporary techniques.

Bleeding remote from the access site can also produce a forearm hematoma. The most common cause is perforation of a small branch with a guidewire in patients receiving platelet glycoprotein IIb/IIIa inhibitors. When bleeding is identified, hemostasis can be achieved with an Ace bandage or a blood pressure sphygmomanometer. In select cases, the interventional guiding catheter can be placed across the perforation and will produce effective hemostasis.[21]

The bulk of these complications have been minimized with designed radial artery equipment including hydrophilic sheaths, as well as the use of intra-arterial vasodilators like nitroglycerin and verapamil, with possible use of heparin.

Practical Pearls

- Heparin (2–5 K units), verapamil (250 µg), and nitroglycerin (250 µg) introduced into the sheath reduce the complication rate.
- Use of hydrophilic sheaths is important to reduce complication risk.
- Maintain a low threshold for producing a fluoroscopic roadmap of arterial supply of the arm, to reduce risk of arterial puncture.
- Use hydrophilic wires to introduce sheath and catheters.

Conclusion

Complications after PCI, although rare, must be identified early and appropriately dealt with. Failure to recognize the complication and deal with it early in its course may lead to major problems, including fatality. This chapter provides a methodical approach to the management of several complications after PCI.

References

1. Al Suwaidi J, Berger PB, Holmes DR, Jr. Coronary artery stents. *JAMA.* 2000;284(14):1828-1836.

2. Brilakis ES, Best PJ, Elesber AA, et al. Incidence, retrieval methods, and outcomes of stent loss during percutaneous coronary intervention: a large single-center experience. *Catheter Cardiovasc Interv.* 2005;66(3):333-340.

3. Eggebrecht H, Haude M, von Birgelen C, et al. Nonsurgical retrieval of embolized coronary stents. *Catheter Cardiovasc Interv.* 2000;51(4):432-440.

4. Veldhuijzen FL, Bonnier HJ, Michels HR, el Gamal MI, van Gelder BM. Retrieval of undeployed stents from the right coronary artery: report of two cases. *Cathet Cardiovasc Diagn.* 1993;30(3):245-248.

5. Elsner M, Peifer A, Kasper W. Intracoronary loss of balloon-mounted stents: Successful retrieval with a 2 mm-"Microsnare"-device. *Cathet Cardiovasc Diagn.* 1996;39(3):271-276.

6. Foster-Smith KW, Garratt KN, Higano ST, Holmes DR, Jr. Retrieval techniques for managing flexible intracoronary stent misplacement. *Cathet Cardiovasc Diagn.* 1993;30(1):63-68.

7. Douard H, Besse P, Broustet JP. Successful retrieval of a lost coronary stent from the descending aorta using a loop basket intravascular retriever set. *Cathet Cardiovasc Diagn.* 1998;44(2):224-226.

8. Ellis SG, Ajluni S, Arnold AZ, et al. Increased coronary perforation in the new device era. Incidence, classification, management, and outcome. *Circulation.* 1994;90(6):2725-2730.

9. Javaid A, Buch AN, Satler LF, et al. Management and outcomes of coronary artery perforation during percutaneous coronary intervention. *Am J Cardiol.* 2006;98(7):911-914.

10. Gaxiola E, Browne KF. Coronary artery perforation repair using microcoil embolization. *Cathet Cardiovasc Diagn.* 1998;43(4):474-476.

11. Fischell TA, Korban EH, Lauer MA. Successful treatment of distal coronary guidewire-induced perforation with balloon catheter delivery of intracoronary thrombin. *Catheter Cardiovasc Interv.* 2003;58(3):370-374.

12. Tiroch KA, Arora N, Matheny ME, Liu C, Lee TC, Resnic FS. Risk predictors of retroperitoneal hemorrhage following percutaneous coronary intervention. *Am J Cardiol.* 2008;102(11):1473-1476.

13. Farouque HM, Tremmel JA, Raissi Shabari F, et al. Risk factors for the development of retroperitoneal hematoma after percutaneous coronary intervention in the era of glycoprotein IIb/IIIa inhibitors and vascular closure devices. *J Am Coll Cardiol.* 2005;45(3):363-368.

14. Kalapatapu VR, Ali AT, Masroor F, Moursi MM, Eidt JF. Techniques for managing complications of arterial closure devices. *Vasc Endovascular Surg.* 2006;40(5):399-408.

15. Dangas G, Mehran R, Kokolis S, et al. Vascular complications after percutaneous coronary interventions following hemostasis with manual compression versus arteriotomy closure devices. *J Am Coll Cardiol.* 2001;38(3):638-641.

16. Koreny M, Riedmuller E, Nikfardjam M, Siostrzonek P, Mullner M. Arterial puncture closing devices compared with standard manual compression after cardiac catheterization: systematic review and meta-analysis. *JAMA.* 2004; 291(3):350-357.

17. Eikelboom JW, Mehta SR, Anand SS, Xie C, Fox KA, Yusuf S. Adverse impact of bleeding on prognosis in patients with acute coronary syndromes. *Circulation.* 2006;114(8):774-782.

18. Ndrepepa G, Berger PB, Mehilli J, et al. Periprocedural bleeding and 1-year outcome after percutaneous coronary interventions: appropriateness of including bleeding as a component of a quadruple end point. *J Am Coll Cardiol.* 2008;51(7):690-697.

19. Kinnaird TD, Stabile E, Mintz GS, et al. Incidence, predictors, and prognostic implications of bleeding and blood transfusion following percutaneous coronary interventions. *Am J Cardiol.* 2003;92(8):930-935.

20. Agostoni P, Biondi-Zoccai GG, de Benedictis ML, et al. Radial versus femoral approach for percutaneous coronary diagnostic and interventional procedures: systematic overview and meta-analysis of randomized trials. *J Am Coll Cardiol.* 2004;44(2):349-356.

21. Bazemore E, Mann JT, 3rd. Problems and complications of the transradial approach for coronary interventions: a review. *J Invasive Cardiol.* Mar 2005;17(3):156-159.

Chapter 10

Optimal Long-term Therapy of the Patient after Percutaneous Coronary Intervention

Dharam J. Kumbhani

The early days of percutaneous coronary intervention (PCI) were often limited by restenosis and a high rate of complications, mainly due to a reliance on balloon angioplasty alone and suboptimal adjunctive pharmacotherapy. Stents, as well as potent antiplatelet agents, have enabled PCI to become the mainstay of revascularization in patients with significant coronary artery disease. The advent of drug-eluting stents (DESs) (Fig. 10.1) earlier this decade, in particular, has significantly reduced the incidence of restenosis, the Achilles heel of their predecessors, bare metal stents (BMSs). However, DESs have been found to be associated with a small, but significantly increased risk of late stent thrombosis, as compared with BMSs.[1] The risk of in-stent restenosis thus needs to be balanced against a risk of stent thrombosis in every patient.[2,3] This risk–benefit analysis guides the decision regarding the type of stent to be used for PCI in almost all patients, which in turn dictates the optimal duration of antiplatelet therapy in these patients.

Overview of Antiplatelet Agents Post Intervention

Given the central role that platelets play in atherothrombosis, as well as in thrombosis following PCI, antiplatelet agents play a pivotal role in the management of patients during and after PCI. Currently used antiplatelet agents for long-term therapy post-PCI include aspirin, thienopyridines, and others such as cilostazol. Several newer agents are also currently being investigated. The cornerstone of therapy post-PCI is dual antiplatelet therapy—aspirin, along with a thienopyridine (currently clopidogrel), owing to their synergistic actions on platelet activity.

Aspirin

Aspirin, or acetyl salicylic acid (ASA), is the most widely used and cost-effective drug in the prevention of platelet aggregation. It exerts its antiplatelet action

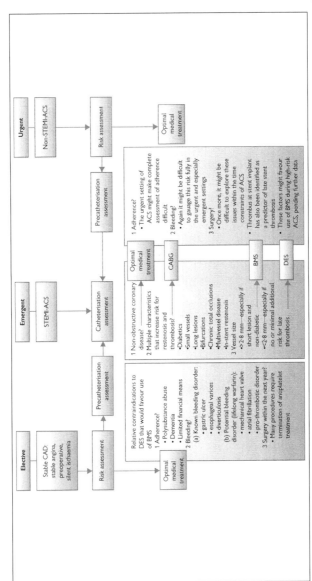

Figure 10.1 Suggested approach for use of drug-eluting stents to boost benefit and reduce harm. ACS, acute coronary syndrome; BMS, bare-metal stent; CAD, coronary artery disease; CABG, coronary artery bypass grafting; DES, drug-eluting stent; STEMI, ST elevation myocardial infarction. Adapted from Bavry AA, Bhatt DL. Appropriate use of drug-eluting stents: balancing the reduction in restenosis with the concern of late thrombosis. *Lancet.* 2008;371:2124-2143, with permission of the publisher (Elsevier).

mainly by irreversibly acetylating a serine residue of platelet cyclooxygenase (COX)-1,[4] thus inhibiting the formation of thromboxane A2, which is a potent stimulator of platelets.

Currently, the American College of Cardiology/American Heart Association (ACC/AHA) recommends that, after PCI, in patients without allergy or increased risk of bleeding, aspirin (162–325 mg daily) should be given for at least 1 month after BMS implantation, 3 months after sirolimus-eluting stent implantation, and 6 months after paclitaxel-eluting stent implantation, after which daily long-term aspirin use should be continued indefinitely at a dose of 75–162 mg (Class I, level of evidence: B).[5] This dose achieves an efficacy that is comparable to higher doses, but without a significant increase in bleeding or gastrointestinal toxicity.[6] In patients for whom the physician is concerned about risk of bleeding, a lower dose of 75–162 mg of aspirin is reasonable during the initial period after stent implantation (Class IIa, level of evidence: C).[5]

Thienopyridines

Thienopyridines exert their antiplatelet effects by irreversibly blocking the $P2Y_{12}$ receptor, thereby inhibiting platelet activation through adenosine diphosphate (ADP).[7] Currently, clopidogrel is the most widely used thienopyridine.

Ticlopidine

Ticlopidine is converted to its active metabolite in vivo. Data regarding the use of ticlopidine 250 mg twice daily as dual antiplatelet therapy along with aspirin following PCI are available mainly for BMS PCI.[8] However, the association of ticlopidine with hypercholesterolemia and hematologic dyscrasias, often severe, have led to a virtual abandonment of this therapy as an alternative to aspirin or clopidogrel in most situations.

According to the ACC/AHA, ticlopidine is currently recommended only in patients who are allergic to clopidogrel (in the absence of contraindications).

Clopidogrel

Clopidogrel is a prodrug, and it is converted to its active metabolite in the liver. Dual therapy with aspirin and clopidogrel is currently the mainstay in the management of patients undergoing PCI.

The optimal duration of long-term therapy with clopidogrel is currently unknown. When DESs were initially approved by the U.S. Food and Drug Administration (FDA) in 2003, dual antiplatelet therapy with aspirin and clopidogrel was recommended for 3 months following sirolimus-eluting stent implantation, and for 6 months following paclitaxel-eluting stent implantation. Given reports of late and very late stent thrombosis in patients receiving a DES compared with BMS, dual antiplatelet therapy is currently recommended for at least 12 months in these patients.[1,9]

Although conventionally a daily dose of 75 mg is utilized as maintenance therapy, recent data seem to suggest that a higher dose of 150 mg daily achieves greater platelet inhibition.[10] Moreover, single-center studies have indicated that this strategy is associated with better clinical outcomes at 30 days, especially after DES implantation.[11] This strategy is, however, not recommended for all patients, and can be considered in patients at high risk of stent thrombosis, such as in those with demonstrated antiplatelet resistance. In addition, chronic long-term therapy with clopidogrel may not achieve adequate platelet inhibition prior to PCI. A loading dose of 300–600 mg is usually readministered in this setting.[12]

Current ACC/AHA recommendation for all post-PCI stented patients receiving a DES, is that clopidogrel 75 mg daily should be given for at least 12 months if patients are not at high risk of bleeding. For post-PCI patients receiving a BMS, clopidogrel should be given for a minimum of 1 month and ideally up to 12 months (unless the patient is at increased risk of bleeding; then it should be given for a minimum of 2 weeks) (Class I, level of evidence: B). Continuation of clopidogrel therapy beyond 1 year may be considered in patients undergoing DES placement (Class IIb, level of evidence: C).[5] In patients in whom subacute thrombosis may be catastrophic or lethal (unprotected left main, bifurcating left main, or last patent coronary vessel), platelet aggregation studies may be considered, and the dose of clopidogrel increased to 150 mg/day if less than 50% inhibition of platelet aggregation is demonstrated (Class IIb, level of evidence: C).[13]

Prasugrel

Prasugrel is a newer-generation thienopyridine that, like clopidogrel, is a prodrug that is converted to an active metabolite in vivo. However, it results in more rapid, higher, and more consistent levels of platelet inhibition than does clopidogrel, with significantly less variation in individual response.[14,15] Prasugrel at a 60 mg loading dose followed by 10 mg daily was recently shown to be associated with a significant clinical benefit, albeit with a higher risk of bleeding, as compared with a 300 mg loading dose followed by 75 mg daily of clopidogrel in patients presenting with acute coronary syndromes.[16] Prasugrel was approved by the FDA earlier this year, and it is likely to figure prominently in future PCI management guidelines.

Antiplatelet Drug Resistance

Antiplatelet drug resistance refers to the development of a thrombotic event while on antiplatelet agents due to ineffective or incomplete platelet inhibition. Low levels of platelet inhibition have also been associated with an elevated risk of ischemic events.[17] Although probably best characterized for aspirin, "resistance" or "hypo-responsiveness" has also been described for clopidogrel and GP IIb/IIIa inhibitors.[18] Although "resistance" may in fact result from patient noncompliance, a number of mechanisms for true antiplatelet resistance have been elucidated (Table 10.1). Although not currently recommended for routine use, a number of platelet function tests are being evaluated,[18,19] and some assays have demonstrated exciting initial clinical results.[20] Further large-scale randomized studies of this and other assays will help clarify their role in routine medical practice.

Other Agents

Cilostazol

Cilostazol exerts its antiplatelet action by selective antagonism of the phosphodiesterase (PDE) 3A enzyme. In addition, it also inhibits the uptake of adenosine,

Table 10.1 Possible mechanisms of antiplatelet resistance

- Bioavailability
  - Noncompliance
  - Under-dosing
  - Poor absorption (enteric-coated aspirin)
  - Interference
    —NSAID coadministration (competes with aspirin for serine 530 of COX-1)
    —Atorvastatin (interferes with cytochrome P450-mediated metabolism of clopidogrel)
- Platelet function
  - Incomplete suppression of thromboxane A2 generation (aspirin)
  - Accelerated platelet turnover, with introduction into bloodstream of newly formed, drug-unaffected platelets
  - Stress-induced COX-2 in platelets (aspirin)
  - Increased platelet sensitivity to ADP and collagen
- Single-nucleotide polymorphisms
  - Receptors: P2Y12 H2 haplotype (clopidogrel), GP IIb/IIIa, collagen receptor, thromboxane receptor, etc.
  - Enzymes: COX-1, COX-2, thromboxane A2 synthase, etc. (aspirin)
- Platelet interactions with other blood cells
  - Endothelial cells and monocytes provide PGH_2 to platelets (bypassing COX-1) and synthesize their own thromboxane A2 (aspirin)
- Other factors
  - Smoking
  - Hypercholesterolemia
  - Obesity (? elevated fibrinogen)
  - Diabetes (? elevated fibrinogen)

ADP, adenosine diphosphate; COX, cyclooxygenase; NSAID, nonsteroidal anti-inflammatory drug.

Adapted from Michelson AD. Platelet function testing in cardiovascular diseases. *Circulation.* 2004; 110:e489-493. Copyright © 2004, American Heart Association, Inc. With permission from Wolters Kluwer Health.

and has been shown to inhibit platelet aggregation. Most, if not all, of its actions are mediated by cyclic adenosine monophosphate (cAMP).[21] Cilostazol (200 mg daily) has been extensively evaluated as an alternative to thienopyridines in patients undergoing PCI, and it may be effective in reducing restenosis and repeat revascularization.[22] Recently, cilostazol has been evaluated as triple antiplatelet therapy, in addition to aspirin and clopidogrel, in patients undergoing DES PCI, and it has been shown to be associated with superior intermediate-term clinical outcomes.[23] Given lack of long-term and placebo-controlled data, cilostazol does not figure in current ACC/AHA PCI guidelines.

Need for Warfarin

Patients with conditions such as mechanical heart valves, chronic atrial fibrillation, and venous thromboembolism are required to be on warfarin, a vitamin

K antagonist, sometimes lifelong. When such patients undergo PCI and need dual antiplatelet therapy, they have a significantly higher risk of major and minor bleeding, which can be as high as 6.6% and 14.9%, respectively.[24] Discontinuation of warfarin might increase the potential for stroke, whereas discontinuation of clopidogrel might result in increased risk for stent thrombosis; both events are associated with significant morbidity and mortality. Consideration for preferential BMS PCI should thus be made in patients needing chronic anticoagulation, to minimize the duration of triple therapy as much as possible.[3]

Need for Noncardiac Surgery or Other Invasive Procedures While on Dual Antiplatelet Therapy

Noncardiac surgery and most invasive procedures can increase the risk of stent thrombosis, especially when the procedure is performed early after stent implantation. Factors include incomplete/nonendothelialization of the stent, the inflammatory milieu associated with surgery, and premature cessation of dual antiplatelet therapy. Aspirin and thienopyridines need to be discontinued for at least 5–7 days prior to surgery to restore normal hemostasis. A number of strategies to minimize the risk of perioperative stent thrombosis are outlined in the Practical Pearls section.[25,26]

Practical Pearls

- *Delay the procedure as long as possible*: Unnecessary and nonemergent procedures, which can safely be performed after the minimum duration of recommended dual antiplatelet therapy has been completed (6 weeks after BMS PCI and 12 months after DES PCI), should be delayed.

- *Continue antiplatelet therapy during the perioperative period*: Some surgeries, such as cataract removal, routine dermatological surgeries, and dental extractions can be safely completed with the patient on aspirin and clopidogrel, without significantly increasing surgical bleeding. Some other more invasive procedures can be similarly safely conducted with the patient on low-dose aspirin. Dual antiplatelet therapy should be resumed as soon as 24 hours or the next day after most surgeries, if possible. Some authorities recommend reloading with 600 mg of clopidogrel in patients with such interruptions in antiplatelet therapy, although this approach has not been validated in clinical studies.

- *Avoid preoperative revascularization*: Most patients with stable coronary disease needing noncardiac surgery do not necessarily benefit from preoperative revascularization. Only patients with unstable coronary syndromes or high-risk features should be considered for revascularization.[27] A recent consideration has been the use of balloon angioplasty alone in patients needing semi-emergent surgery and having high-risk coronary disease. Percutaneous coronary intervention with stents can be performed after surgery if indicated.

- *Stent selection*: If a patient is expected to need noncardiac surgery within 1 year, it is best to use BMS when possible.

- *Bridging therapy*: If there is a need for an invasive procedure before dual anti-platelet therapy can be safely stopped, one approach is to bridge patients with a glycoprotein IIb/IIIa inhibitor, with or without heparin, in the perioperative period, before antiplatelet therapy can be resumed. This approach has not been validated in clinical trials.

References

1. Bavry AA, Kumbhani DJ, Helton TJ, Borek PP, Mood GR, Bhatt DL. Late thrombosis of drug-eluting stents: a meta-analysis of randomized clinical trials. *Am J Med.* 2006;119:1056-1061.

2. Kumbhani DJ, Bavry AA, Bhatt DL. Late stent thrombosis with drug-eluting stents: the price to pay to prevent restenosis? *Indian Heart J.* 2007;59:B113-117.

3. Bavry AA, Bhatt DL. Appropriate use of drug-eluting stents: balancing the reduction in restenosis with the concern of late thrombosis. *Lancet.* 2008; 371:2134-2143.

4. Roth GJ, Stanford N, Majerus PW. Acetylation of prostaglandin synthase by aspirin. *Proc Natl Acad Sci U S A.* 1975;72:3073-3076.

5. King SB, 3rd, Smith SC, Jr., Hirshfeld JW, Jr., et al. 2007 focused update of the ACC/AHA/SCAI 2005 guideline update for percutaneous coronary intervention: a report of the American College of Cardiology/American Heart Association Task Force on Practice guidelines. *J Am Coll Cardiol.* 2008;51:172-209.

6. Collaborative meta-analysis of randomised trials of antiplatelet therapy for prevention of death, myocardial infarction, and stroke in high risk patients. *BMJ.* 2002;324:71-86.

7. Kumbhani DJ, Bhatt DL. Use of oral antiplatelet agents in acute coronary syndromes. *Arch Med Sci.* 2009;in press.

8. Leon MB, Baim DS, Popma JJ, et al. A clinical trial comparing three antithrombotic-drug regimens after coronary-artery stenting. Stent Anticoagulation Restenosis Study Investigators. *N Engl J Med.* 1998;339:1665-1671.

9. Eisenstein EL, Anstrom KJ, Kong DF, et al. Clopidogrel use and long-term clinical outcomes after drug-eluting stent implantation. *JAMA.* 2007;297:159-168.

10. von Beckerath N, Kastrati A, Wieczorek A, et al. A double-blind, randomized study on platelet aggregation in patients treated with a daily dose of 150 or 75 mg of clopidogrel for 30 days. *Eur Heart J.* 2007;28:1814-1819.

11. Han YL, Wang B, Li Y, et al. A high maintenance dose of clopidogrel improves short-term clinical outcomes in patients with acute coronary syndrome undergoing drug-eluting stent implantation. *Chin Med J (Engl).* 2009;122:793-797.

12. Kastrati A, von Beckerath N, Joost A, et al. Loading with 600 mg clopidogrel in patients with coronary artery disease with and without chronic clopidogrel therapy. *Circulation.* 2004;110:1916-1919.

13. Smith SC, Jr., Feldman TE, Hirshfeld JW, Jr., et al. ACC/AHA/SCAI 2005 guideline update for percutaneous coronary intervention: a report of the American College of Cardiology/American Heart Association Task Force on Practice

Guidelines (ACC/AHA/SCAI Writing Committee to Update 2001 Guidelines for Percutaneous Coronary Intervention). *Circulation.* 2006;113:e166-286.

14. Brandt JT, Payne CD, Wiviott SD, et al. A comparison of prasugrel and clopidogrel loading doses on platelet function: magnitude of platelet inhibition is related to active metabolite formation. *Am Heart J.* 2007;153:66e9-16.

15. Wiviott SD, Trenk D, Frelinger AL, et al. Prasugrel compared with high loading- and maintenance-dose clopidogrel in patients with planned percutaneous coronary intervention: The Prasugrel in Comparison to Clopidogrel for Inhibition of Platelet Activation and Aggregation-Thrombolysis in Myocardial Infarction 44 trial. *Circulation.* 2007;116:2923-2932.

16. Wiviott SD, Braunwald E, McCabe CH, et al. Prasugrel versus clopidogrel in patients with acute coronary syndromes. *N Engl J Med.* 2007;357:2001-2015.

17. Price MJ, Endemann S, Gollapudi RR, et al. Prognostic significance of post-clopidogrel platelet reactivity assessed by a point-of-care assay on thrombotic events after drug-eluting stent implantation. *Eur Heart J.* 2008;29:992-1000.

18. Michelson AD. Platelet function testing in cardiovascular diseases. *Circulation.* 2004;110:e489-493.

19. Bhatt DL. What makes platelets angry: diabetes, fibrinogen, obesity, and impaired response to antiplatelet therapy? *J Am Coll Cardiol.* 2008;52:1060-1061.

20. Aleil B, Jacquemin L, De Poli F, et al. Clopidogrel 150 mg/day to overcome low responsiveness in patients undergoing elective percutaneous coronary intervention: Results from the VASP-02 (Vasodilator-Stimulated Phosphoprotein-02) randomized study. *JACC Cardiovasc Interv.* 2008;1:631-638.

21. Schror K. The pharmacology of cilostazol. *Diabetes Obes Metab.* 2002;4(Suppl 2):S14-19.

22. Biondi-Zoccai GG, Lotrionte M, Anselmino M, et al. Systematic review and meta-analysis of randomized clinical trials appraising the impact of cilostazol after percutaneous coronary intervention. *Am Heart J.* 2008;155:1081-1089.

23. Chen KY, Rha SW, Li YJ, et al. Triple versus dual antiplatelet therapy in patients with acute ST-segment elevation myocardial infarction undergoing primary percutaneous coronary intervention. *Circulation.* 2009;119:3207-3214.

24. Khurram Z, Chou E, Minutello R, et al. Combination therapy with aspirin, clopidogrel and warfarin following coronary stenting is associated with a significant risk of bleeding. *J Invasive Cardiol.* 2006;18:162-164.

25. Brilakis ES, Banerjee S, Berger PB. Perioperative management of patients with coronary stents. *J Am Coll Cardiol.* 2007;49:2145-2150.

26. Grines CL, Bonow RO, Casey DE, Jr., et al. Prevention of premature discontinuation of dual antiplatelet therapy in patients with coronary artery stents: a science advisory from the American Heart Association, American College of Cardiology, Society for Cardiovascular Angiography and Interventions, American College of Surgeons, and American Dental Association, with representation from the American College of Physicians. *Circulation.* 2007;115:813-818.

27. McFalls EO, Ward HB, Moritz TE, et al. Coronary-artery revascularization before elective major vascular surgery. *N Engl J Med.* 2004;351:2795-2804.

Chapter 11

Noncoronary
Interventions

Chapter 11a

Renal and Mesenteric Artery Interventions

On Topaz, Allyne Topaz, and Pritam R. Polkampally

Interventions for Renal Artery Stenosis

Atherosclerotic renal artery stenosis (RAS) accounts for impaired perfusion and adverse clinical sequelae.[1] A majority (>90%) of renal arterial obstructions in adults are caused by atherosclerotic vascular disease.[2] Left untreated, RAS may cause renal atrophy and subsequent need for permanent dialysis, uncontrolled hypertension, and severe congestive heart failure (CHF). Over the last decade, a dramatic paradigm shift in the treatment of RAS took place. Vascular surgery was replaced as the preferred treatment for RAS initially by percutaneous transluminal angioplasty (PTA) and subsequently by percutaneous transluminal angioplasty with stenting (PTAS). Noninvasive diagnostic methods such as magnetic resonance angiography (MRA), computed tomography angiography (CTA), and duplex ultrasonography are highly beneficial, but none have obviated the role of the "gold standard," renal arteriography.[2]

Clinical Considerations

Patients with RAS may present with hypertension, failure to control blood pressure with multidrug therapy, renal dysfunction following administration of angiotensin-converting enzyme (ACE)-inhibitor or contrast, CHF, and flash pulmonary edema. Percutaneous transluminal angioplasty with stenting of RAS achieves a 95%–98% technical success rate, with less than 5% major complications and 10% restenosis.[3] However, despite the marked advances offered by PTAS, this modality is not universally accepted.[4–6] Enrollment in ongoing clinical studies (e.g., CORAL) is considerably low, and unrealistic expectations for PTAS outcome prevail. Completed studies comparing medical therapy to balloon angioplasty for treatment of hypertension[7] allowed a large proportion of the patients who failed medical therapy to cross over to the angioplasty treatment. Other randomized investigations of stenting versus medical therapy[8] included lesions of less than 70%, failed to stent a large number of those patients who were randomized to stenting,[8,9] or set arbitrary resistive renal indices to determine procedural success.[9] An unacceptably high rate of technical failures, vascular complications,[8] and "disappointing PTAS results"[8–11] have also been reported. In reality, the combined deleterious effects of coexisting atherosclerosis, hypertension, and diabetes frequently causes permanent damage to kidney function before PTAS. Yet the only component that can still be modified is the compromised flow secondary to RAS. In these instances, PTAS or bypass surgery may preserve some or even all residual renal function.[10] Regrettably, the absence of "angina renalis" and the unavailability of precise tests to detect silent ischemic kidney creates a "permissive" clinical tolerance for impaired renal function, despite the grave risk of kidney loss and resultant permanent dialysis. Renal artery stenosis should be particularly suspected in patients with accelerated hypertension (sudden and persistent worsening of previously controlled hypertension), resistant hypertension (failure to achieve goal blood pressure in patients who are adhering to full doses of an appropriate three-drug regimen that includes a diuretic), or malignant hypertension (hypertension with coexistent evidence of acute end-organ damage, such as acute renal failure, acutely decompensated congestive heart failure, new visual or neurological disturbance, and/or advanced [grade III/IV] retinopathy).[12]

Management of the Patient with Renal Artery Stenosis

Case Selection

The indications for PTAS for treatment of significant RAS include hemodynamically significant RAS associated with accelerated hypertension; resistant hypertension; malignant hypertension; hypertension with an unexplained unilateral small kidney; hypertension with intolerance to medication; asymptomatic bilateral or solitary viable kidney; bilateral RAS and progressive chronic kidney disease; recurrent, unexplained congestive heart failure or sudden, unexplained pulmonary edema; RAS in a patient who requires treatment with ACE inhibitors for retinopathy and nephropathy; and renal transplant with an arterial stenosis or renal bypass graft stenosis producing hypertension, azotemia, or both.[13,14] However, the only American College of Cardiology/American Heart Association (ACC/AHA) Class I recommendation for percutaneous revascularization is significant RAS with recurrent and unexplained CHF or pulmonary edema.

An important goal for PTAS of RAS is to eliminate the significant transstenosis pressure gradient. Most recently, Leesar et al. reported that the best criteria for prediction of hypertension improvement after stenting of RAS is a hyperemic systolic gradient of 21 mm Hg or higher.[15]

From pathologic and clinical perspectives, the ominous rapid progression of severe RAS toward total occlusion and resultant permanent kidney loss is of major concern. Even a moderate angiographic stenosis of 50%–60% is associated with a 11.7% cumulative incidence of renal atrophy and a 28% cumulative incidence of disease progression over 2-year period.[16] Thus, critical RAS cases may be considered for PTAS to remove the danger of impending renal artery closure (Fig. 11a.1a,b).

Technical Aspects of Renal Percutaneous Transluminal Angioplasty

Vascular access can be obtained by a femoral, brachial, or radial approach. Adjunct pharmacotherapy includes aspirin, heparin (target ACT 225–250),

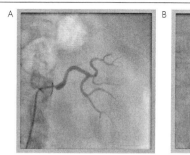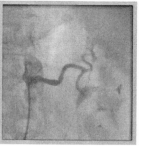

Figure 11a.1 Renal artery stenosis. (A) A patient with uncontrolled hypertension, CHF and unstable angina. Bilateral critical renal artery stenosis was found. Angiogram of the critical ostial left renal artery stenosis is depicted. (B) Results post debulking and adjunct stenting. The patient's clinical condition improved dramatically post intervention.

and clopidogrel, either before or immediately post stenting.[17] A direct thrombin inhibitor instead of heparin can be used, with dose adjustment for renal function, although this line of treatment is not as well studied. A protection protocol for contrast-induced nephropathy using acetylcysteine (Mucomyst) 1,200 mg b.i.d. administered intravenously or orally) is indicated regardless of the baseline creatinine. Plavix is administered for at least 1 month post renal intervention.

The most important technical issues of renal PTAS relate to safety of equipment manipulation and to the crucial limitations on the volume of hazardous contrast medium.[18] Targeted renal therapy by direct infusion of the short-acting selective dopamine 1 agonist vasodilator Fenoldopam through dedicated renal catheters has been studied.[19] Most commonly a 6 or 8 Fr short left internal mammary artery (LIMA) guiding catheter is used over a 0.035- or 0.014-inch guidewire. Other useful guiding catheters include renal curve, multipurpose (mainly for brachial approach), Simmons Sidewinder, Sos Omni, Cobra, and Judkins right coronary. The guiding catheter is flushed frequently to avoid accumulation of any atherosclerotic or thrombotic material. Then the ostium of the renal artery is gently engaged and an adequate pressure wave form should be verified. A cross-lesion gradient can be recorded either by a pull-back technique with the guide catheter or with insertion of a pressure wire. A selective angiogram is performed in anteroposterior (AP) view with peripheral magnification and, if indicated, shallow left anterior oblique (LAO) and right anterior oblique (RAO) projections are obtained. The angiographic injections should contain a 50/50 mixture of contrast media and saline. We prefer to cross the lesion with a 0.014-inch SpartaCore (Abbott Vascular, Santa Clara, CA) guidewire. Other available guidewires are the 0.035-inch Wholey Hi-Torque J (Mallinckrodt, St. Louis, MO) or the Zipwire 0.035-inch (Boston Scientific, Natick, MA). In instances when a guidewire needs enhanced support, we cross with a 0.014-inch guidewire and exchange it through an exchange catheter system (Quick Cross, Spectranetics,

Colorado Springs, CO) with a stiff, supportive Platinum Plus guidewire. It is crucial that the guidewire is held firmly throughout the entire procedure with the tip positioned at a large tributary of the main renal artery. This is required to avoid distal migration of the guidewire into the renal parenchyma, with catastrophic sequelae. For further determination of the target lesion and the characteristics of the target vessel, a rapid-exchange intra-renal ultrasound (Volcano Technologies, Rancho Cordova, CA) may be undertaken, but it is rarely used in clinical practice. The incorporation of a filter protection system is a controversial topic. Operators who are concerned with the danger of distal embolization from the target plaque favor deployment of a protective system in every renal intervention.[20–22] However, the available embolic protection devices are not specifically designed for use in renal arteries, and there are legitimate concerns about the floppy-tip guidewires of the protection systems, incompatibility with the limited landing zone, difficult delivery, and kinking upon the retrieval of the filter.[23] In practice, few operators use an emboli protection device.

When treating severe-critical RAS (defined as >90%, with a gradient of >50 mm Hg), especially in lesions exhibiting a markedly eccentric plaque and associated thrombus, debulking is an option.[24] This facilitates subsequent balloon and stent deployment. Among available peripheral balloons are the Aviator (Cordis, Raden, Netherlands), Prolifer (AngioDynamics, Queensburg, NY), and Agil Trac (Abbott Vascular, Santa Clara, CA). For balloon deployment, we apply a unique technique that takes into consideration the sharp aortic exit angle of the renal arteries with the corresponding retroperitoneal "free suspension." Thus, in the absence of surrounding supportive tissue around these vessels, radial balloon distension pressures are distributed to the entire circumference of the vessel without any counter vectors. Consequently, arterial wall damage in the form of dissections and even perforations may rarely occur during renal angioplasty. Plaque disintegration and distal embolization of atherosclerotic debris may also accompany the balloon inflations as well.[20] Thus, we perform a soft molding inflation applying a very low pressure. For example, a balloon with a nominal pressure of 10 atm is inflated to 1–2 atm only. In our experience, in most instances, this technique achieves adequate changes in the plaque's morphology, eliminates dissections and perforations, reduces distal embolization, and facilitates stenting. For lesions that require a semi-compliant balloon, either the NanoCross or the EverCross balloons (eV3, Plymouth, MN) are useful. In cases with a very resistant target lesion that requires a high-pressure inflation, the Conquest (Bard Vascular, Tempe, AZ) high-pressure balloon (rated burst pressure 30 atm) can be applied. The renal stents utilized should be based on an expandable balloon platform and deployed up to nominal pressure. Among commonly used stents are the Genesis (Cordis, Raden, Netherlands) and the Paramount Mini (eV3, Plymouth, MN). Importantly, the stent size should precisely match the normal caliber of the artery and not the segment containing a poststenotic dilatation. Along the stent deployment, the guiding catheter is gently pushed forward in order to slightly elevate the ostial-proximal portion of the stent. This maneuver places the stent in a perfect adaptation to the vessel's natural anatomic course. For ostial narrowing, the stent should cover the entire ostium, bulging 1–2 mm into the aorta. Repeat ultrasound for verification of adequate stent expansion may be useful. This should be followed by documentation of the postprocedural residual gradient. Upon completion of the renal PTAS, a normal flow in the targeted renal artery should be present. Postprocedural care includes aspirin for life and clopidogrel for at least 1 month. Close follow-up of renal function is mandatory.

Interventions for Mesenteric Ischemia

Acute and chronic mesenteric ischemia are caused by atherosclerotic/thrombotic disease, arterial embolic occlusive disease, dissection, vasculitis, median arcuate ligament, low flow state secondary to myocardial infarction, severe CHF, and sepsis. The pathophysiology of acute and chronic mesenteric ischemia relates to disease in the three major aortic branches that provide gastrointestinal blood supply: the celiac artery, superior mesenteric artery, and inferior mesenteric artery.[25] Most atherosclerotic lesions involve the ostium or the proximal 3 cm of a mesenteric artery. The indications for mesenteric artery intervention include chronic mesenteric ischemia (defined as unexplained weight loss with postprandial abdominal pain and chronic nausea, vomiting, diarrhea) with significant stenosis or occlusion of two or more visceral vessels, or acute symptoms in a mesentery artery stenosis (MAS) patient who is not a surgical candidate. The revascularization can involve treatment with transcatheter lytic therapy, balloon angioplasty, and stenting in selected patients (Figs. 11a.2a–c and 11a.3a,b).[25] The advent and convenience of percutaneous techniques for the management of chronic and acute mesenteric ischemia has offered an alternative strategy for a significant number of patients for whom open surgery poses significant risk.[26] For acute mesenteric ischemia, angiography in AP and lateral views is still regarded as the gold standard, yet CTA is an excellent tool as well. Initial diagnosis of chronic mesenteric ischemia should be confirmed by Doppler ultrasonography. A peak velocity of 275 cm/sec or greater represents 70% stenosis (sensitivity 92%, specificity 96%). For PTA, either a femoral or transbrachial approach may be used. Standard medications are heparin, clopidogrel, aspirin, and selective injection of a thrombolytic agent, if indicated. Equipment selection includes a 7 or 8 Fr guide catheter, 0.014- or 0.035-inch guidewires, a low-profile rapid-exchange peripheral balloon, and standard balloon-expandable peripheral stenting, as used in renal PTA (described earlier).[25] Balloon-expandable stents are preferred over self-expandable stents except in selected cases in which external compression on the superior mesenteric artery requires application of self-expandable Nitinol stents. The technical success rate of PTA for MAS is high at 80%–96%, with a major complication rate of 8%–16% and long-term success rates of 67%–83%. The 6-month patency is 92%, and the 18-month patency is 74%.[27] Silva and colleagues reported a 29% restenosis rate among 59 consecutive patients who

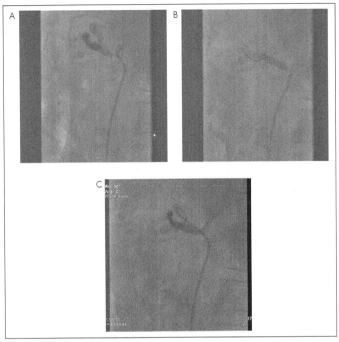

Figure 11a.2 Celiac artery stenosis. (A) 71-year-old male with severe multisystem atherosclerotic vascular disease. The patient presented with food fear, post-prandial abdominal pain and diarrhea. Angiogram demonstrating 90% ostial celiac artery stenosis (*below*), 80% SMA, and 100% IMA occlusion. (B) Intervention with Spartacore guide-wire, PTA 5.0/20 Quantum balloon followed by stenting with Express SD 7.0/19 stent. (C) Final angiographic results post stenting. The patient had marked clinical improvement. (Courtesy of Chris Metzger, MD, Director Cardiac and peripheral Cath Labs, Wellmont Holston Valley Medical Center, Kingsport, TN.)

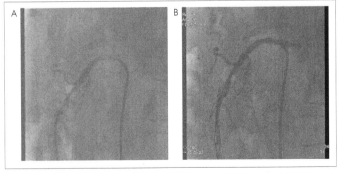

Figure 11a.3 Superior mesenteric artery (SMA) stenosis. (A) Angiogram demonstrating severe ostial stenosis of the SMA. (B) Results after application of balloon and stenting with Express SD 6.0/18 stent. (Courtesy of Chris Metzger, MD, Director Cardiac and peripheral Cath Labs, Wellmont Holston Valley Medical Center, Kingsport, TN.)

underwent stenting for chronic mesenteric ischemia. The restenotic lesions were successfully revascularized through repeat PTA.[27]

Postprocedural care includes aspirin for life and clopidogrel (75 mg/day orally) for at least 1 month. Careful clinical assessment and noninvasive imaging for signs of recurrent mesenteric disease are mandatory. Duplex surveillance should be obtained at 1, 3, and 6 months, and every 6 months thereafter.

Conclusion

- Patients with RAS present with hypertension, failure to control blood pressure with multidrug therapy, renal dysfunction following administration of an ACE inhibitor or contrast, CHF, flash pulmonary edema, and angina.
- Important selection criteria for RAS intervention include severe angiographic stenosis of at least 80% associated with hyperemic systolic gradient 20 mm Hg or greater. Alternatively, a preprocedure peak-to-peak gradient of 25 mm Hg or greater should be present.
- Percutaneous transluminal angioplasty with stenting of RAS achieves a 95%–98% technical success rate, with less than 5% major complications and 10% restenosis.
- Follow-up post PTAS of RAS includes assessment of renal function and modification of cardiovascular risk factors.
- The indications for mesenteric artery intervention include chronic mesenteric ischemia or acute symptoms in a MAS patient who is not a surgical candidate.
- The technical success rate of PTA of MAS is 80%–96%, with a major complication rate of 8%–16%, and long-term success rates of 67%–83%.
- Duplex surveillance should be obtained in 1, 3, and 6 months, and every 6 months thereafter.

Practical Pearls

- Perform the renal angiograms with a 50/50 mixture of contrast and saline to reduce the dye load.
- Administer Mucomyst protocol regardless of baseline creatinine.
- Use a supporting guidewire with soft J-tip configuration.
- Anchor the guidewire during the entire procedure to avoid distal tip migration.
- Deploy soft, molding, compliant balloons with a lower than nominal pressure whenever possible.
- In complex lesions, consider debulking prior to balloon inflation.
- Use balloon-expandable stents.
- Consider intravascular ultrasound for assessment of pre and post balloon dilation and stenting.

References

1. Olin JW, Melia M, Young JR et al. Prevalence of atherosclerotic renal artery stenosis in patients with atherosclerosis elsewhere. *Am J Med.* 1990:88: 46N-51N.

2. Jaff MR. Renal artery duplex ultrasonography. In: Mohler ER, Gerhard-Herman M, Jaff MR, eds. *Essentials of vascular laboratory diagnosis.* New York: Blackwell Futura, 2005:75–83.

3. Safian RD, Hanzel G. Treatment of renal artery stenosis. In: Creager MA, Dzau VJ, Loscalzo J, eds. *Vascular medicine.* Philadelphia: WB Saunders, 2006:349–357.

4. Mukherjee D. Editorial. Renal artery revascularization. Is there a rationale to perform? *J Am Coll Cardiol Intv.* 2009;2:183–184.

5. McLaughlin K, Jardine A, Moss JG. ABC of arterial and venous disease: renal artery stenosis. *BMJ.* 2000:320:1124–1127.

6. Sos TA. The renal stenting debate: is this procedure underused or overused? Yes. *Endovasc Today.* 2006:5:64–68.

7. van Jaarsveld BC, Krijnen P, Pieterman H, et al The effect of balloon angioplasty on hypertension in atherosclerotic renal artery stenosis. Dutch Renal Artery Stenosis Intervention Cooperative Study Group. *N Engl J Med.* 2000:342:1007–1014.

8. Bax L, Wiottez AJ, Kouwenberg HJ, et al. Stent placement in patients with atherosclerotic renal artery stenosis and impaired renal function: a randomized study. *Ann Intern Med.* 2009:150:840–848.

9. Radermacher J, Chavan A, Bleck J, et al. Use of Doppler ultrasonography to predict the outcome of therapy for renal artery stenosis. *N Engl J Med.* 2001:344:410–417.

10. Cooper CJ, Haller ST, Colyer W. Embolic protection and platelet inhibition during renal artery stenting. *Circulation.* 2008:117:2752–2750.

11. Hansen KJ,Cherr GS, Craven TE, et al. Management of ischemic nephropathy: dialysis-free survival after surgical repair. *J Vasc Surg.* 2000:32:472–482.

12. ACC/AHA 2005 Guidelines for the Management of Patients with Peripheral Arterial Disease. *J Am Coll Cardiol.* 2006; 47:1–192.

13. White CJ. Renal artery disease: Facts and myths. *Endovasc Today.* 2003;6:52–58.

14. Olin JW. Renal and mesenteric artery disease. In: Rooke TW, ed. *Vascular medicine and endovascular interventions.* New York: Blackwell Futura, 2007:201–211.

15. Leesar MA, Varma J, Shapira A, et al. Prediction of hypertension improvement after stenting of renal artery stenosis. Comparative accuracy of translesional pressure gradients, intravascular ultrasound, and angiography. *JACC.* 2009:53:2363–2371.

16. Caps MT, Perissinotto C, Zierler RE, et al. Prospective study of atherosclerotic disease progression in the renal artery. *Circulation.* 1998:98:2866–2872.

17. Safian RD, Madder RD. Refining the approach to renal artery revascularization. *JACC Interv.* 2009:2:161–174.

18. Smith J. Tools of the renal trade. *Endovasc Today.* 2006:5:70–71.

19. Allie DE, Weinstock BS, Teirstein P. Targeted renal therapy. *Endovasc Today.* 2006:5;38–42.

20. Henry M, Kionaris C, Henry I, et al. Protected renal stenting with the PercuSurge Guardwire device: a pilot study. *J Endovasc Ther.* 2001:8:227–237.

21. Holden A, Hill A. Renal angioplasty and stenting with distal protection of the main renal artery in ischemic nephropathy. *J Vasc Surg.* 2003:38:762–768.

22. Dubel GJ, Murphy TP. Distal embolic protection for renal arterial interventions. *Cardiovasc Intervent Radiol.* 2007:31:14–22.

23. Dave RM. Renal artery stenting with embolic protection. *Endovasc Today.* 2006:5:43–50.

24. Topaz O, Polkampally PR, Topaz A, et al. Utilization of excimer laser debulking for critical lesions unsuitable for standard renal angioplasty. *Lasers Surg Med.* 2009 Nov;41:622–627.

25. Yazdi HR, Youness F, Laroia S, et al. Mesenteric artery stenting for chronic mesenteric ischemia. *Vasc Dis Mgmt.* 2007;4:180–184.

26. Kasirajan K, O'Hara PJ, Gray BH, et al. Chronic mesenteric ischemia: open surgery versus percutaneous angioplasty and stenting. *J Vasc Surg.* 2001:33:63–71.

27. Silva JA, White CJ, Collins TJ, et al. Endovascular therapy for chronic mesenteric ischemia. *J Am Coll Cardiol.* 2006:47:944–950.

Chapter 11b

Carotid Artery Interventions

Thomas J. Helton

Stroke is the third leading cause of death in the United States, and most occur without warning. At least 5%–12% of strokes occur in patients with carotid disease that is amenable to revascularization. The predominant method of revascularization remains carotid endarterectomy, with 117,000 procedures performed annually; carotid stenting (Fig. 11b.1) is reserved for patients who present high surgical risk (approximately 7,000–10,000 stent procedures are performed annually).[1]

Patient Management

Vascular Access

A successful carotid stenting procedure always begins with appropriate vascular access. Rarely, a right brachial or right radial approach may be necessary to facilitate engagement of an anomalous left carotid originating from the innominate. Contemporary carotid stent delivery systems require either a 6 Fr delivery sheath (also known as a guiding sheath) or an 8 Fr guide catheter system; both have similar internal diameters (0.087–0.090 inches). Operator preference or familiarity often dictates the selection. Operators at our institution typically use the delivery sheath system for the vast majority of carotid interventions; however, the larger guide-based systems offer more support and are useful for tortuous vessels, and in distal or critically tight lesions (Fig. 11b.2).

Carotid Angiography

Aortic arch anatomy is defined by the relationship of the innominate artery to the aortic arch, as well as the origins of the great vessels. Three basic variants of aortic arch anatomy are currently recognized (Fig. 11b.3), and the most common aberration of the great vessels is a "bovine arch" (Fig. 11b.4).

Diagnostic carotid angiography can be performed in nearly all patients with a type 1 or type 2 arch using a JR4 catheter positioned in the common carotid (Table 11b.1). Conversely, a Vitek® or Simmons® catheter JR4 is often needed for a type 3 arch or "bovine" anatomy. Intracranial circulation projections are an essential part of routine carotid angiography, as these images will serve as references should an untoward complication, such as an intracranial embolic event, arise during the intervention.

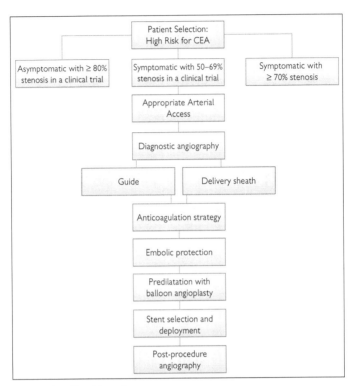

Figure 11b.1 Carotid stenting strategy.

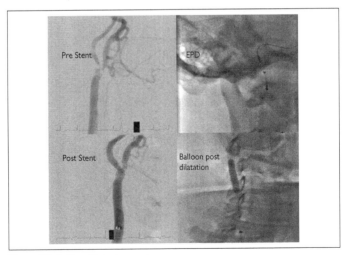

Figure 11b.2 Carotid stent procedure.

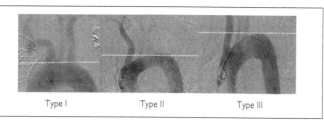

| Type I | Type II | Type III |

Figure 11b.3 Classification of aortic arch type. Type I aortic arch occurs when all three great vessels arise in the same horizontal plane as the outer curvature of the aortic arch. In the type II aortic arch, the innominate arises between the horizontal planes of the outer and inner curvatures of the aortic arch. In the type III aortic arch, the innominate arises below the horizontal plane of the inner curvature of the aortic arch. The degree of difficulty engaging the carotid artery progressively increases from type 1 to type 3 arches.

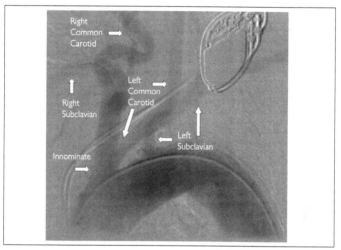

Figure 11b.4 Bovine arch. The bovine arch is the most common arch variant, in which the left common carotid arises as a branch of the innominate artery.

Table 11b.1 Basic carotid angiographic views*

Aortic arch	LAO 30°
Left carotid artery	LAO 30–45°
	Left lateral 90°
Right carotid artery	RAO 30–45°
	Left lateral 90°
Intracranial arteries	PA cranial 20–30°†
	Left lateral 90°

*Supplementary views with contralateral obliques and cranial/caudal angulation may be necessary to better visualize specific lesions or anatomic areas of interest.

†Angulation should be such that the petrous bone is positioned at the base of the orbit.

LAO, left anterior oblique; RAO, right anterior oblique.

Carotid Stenting and Angioplasty

Antithrombotic Strategy

Most operators use heparin 50–70 units/kg bolus to target an activated clotting time (ACT) of 250–300 seconds for carotid interventions, and many give a heparin bolus prior to diagnostic angiography, although after access is obtained.[1] This is typically done on a background of aspirin 325 mg/day and clopidogrel 75 mg/day (after a 300–600 mg loading dose). Post procedure, aspirin should be continued indefinitely and clopidogrel for at least 30 days.[1] The use of bivalirudin was permitted in some carotid stenting trials; however, there are insufficient data to recommend this strategy.[2] The use of low-molecular-weight heparins is neither proven nor recommended during carotid stenting, given the lack of reversibility and long half-lives. Glycoprotein IIb-IIIa inhibitors have not proven useful in this setting and also carry the added potential of increased bleeding.[3]

Guide or Delivery Sheath Engagement

First, the appropriate guiding catheter or delivery sheath must be selected. With a Tuhoy-Borst® adaptor attached to the hub of the guide/delivery sheath, a soft-tip 0.035-inch wire is advanced into the guide/delivery sheath and a diagnostic catheter (JR4) is advanced over the wire. The diagnostic catheter and soft-tip wire are positioned 6–8 cm beyond the tip of the guide/delivery sheath and used to initially engage the left common carotid or innominate artery. The soft-tipped wire is then exchanged for a stiff angle Glidewire®, which is advanced into the external carotid artery. Next, the guide/delivery sheath is slowly advanced over the Glidewire®/diagnostic catheter combination to the distal common carotid.

Embolic Protection

Selection of an embolic protection strategy is the next step. Many types of embolic protection devices (EPDs) exist; however, most of the supporting data for carotid stenting are with filter-type EPDs (Table 11b.2). The filter-type EPDs are a subset of distal protection devices in that they require the lesion to be crossed and the device deployed distal to the lesion. Occasionally, the lesion has to be predilated to allow passage of the filter. Filter devices typically come with a soft-tipped 0.014-inch wire that is advanced distal to the lesion to the cervical portion of the internal carotid artery. This area, just proximal to the petrous segment, is typically the ideal landing zone for distal EPDs, as it is usually straight and devoid of significant atherosclerotic plaque.[4] Once positioned correctly (advanced over the wire in a closed or sheathed position), the filter device is deployed by advancing the filter out of its integrated sheath.

Balloon Angioplasty/Stenting

Predilation with a 4.0 × 20 mm balloon is often performed to allow passage of the stent across the lesion.[4] Carotid stents come in two basic configurations: tapered and nontapered. Tapered stents are ideally suited for lesions that start in a larger vessel (i.e., the distal common carotid) and extend into a smaller

Table 11b.2 Embolic protection devices[1,4,5]

Device Type	Advantages	Disadvantages
Distal protection with filter device	• Preservation of antegrade flow • Permits contrast imaging during procedure • Ease of use	• Incomplete debris capture • Filter clogging • Debris loss during device retrieval • May require lesion pre dilatation for delivery • May be difficult to retrieve across stent
Distal protection with balloon occlusion	• Ease of use • Near complete debris capture with both large and small particles	• No antegrade flow • No contrast imaging during procedure • Balloon induced vessel trauma • Movement or inadequate apposition during procedure
Proximal protection with balloon occlusion	• Eliminates guidewire attributable embolization • Operator selects guidewire • Retrograde distal internal carotid flow	• No antegrade flow • Relatively difficult to use, large profile • Static contrast imaging during procedure

Adapted from Bates ER, Babb JD, Casey DE, Jr., et al. ACCF/SCAI/SVMB/SIR/ASITN 2007 Clinical Expert Consensus Document on carotid stenting. *Vasc Med.* 2007;12(1):35-83, with permission of the publisher.

Table 11b.3 Stent design: Advantages and disadvantages[4,5]

Open-Cell		Closed-Cell	
Advantage	Disadvantage	Advantage	Disadvantage
Improved flexibility in tortuous vessels	Difficulty with introducing and retrieving devices	Improved device deliverability and retrieval	Not as flexible in tortuous vessels
Enhanced vessel wall apposition	Protrusion of plaque or thrombus into the vessel lumen	Improved plaque and thrombus coverage with more uniform scaffolding	Relatively less uniform wall apposition
	Separation and protrusion of stent struts and segments	No protruding stent struts	

vessel (i.e., the internal carotid artery). Conversely, nontapered or cylindrical stents are optimally suited for lesions contained within a vessel of uniform size. These stents are either balloon-expandable stainless steel or self-expanding nitinol stents with an open- or closed-cell design, each having unique advantages and disadvantages (Table 11b.3).[5] The vast majority of stents currently used for carotid stenting are nitinol self-expanding stents (Table 11b.4).[5]

Table 11b.4 Currently available carotid stents[1,5]

Stent	Straight		Tapered		Cell Design	Stent Type
	Diameter (mm)	Length (mm)	Diameter (mm)	Length (mm)		
Acculink (Guidant)	5, 6, 7, 8, 9, 10	20, 30, 40	8–6 10–7	20, 30, 40 20, 30, 40	Open	N
Exponent (Medtronic)	6, 7, 8, 9, 10	20, 30, 40	NA	NA	Open	N
Precise (Cordis)	5, 6, 7, 8, 9, 10	30, 40	8–6 9–7 10–8	20, 30, 40 20, 30, 40 20, 30, 40	Open	N
Protégé (EV3)	6, 7, 8, 9, 10	20, 30, 40, 60	8–6 10–7	30, 40	Open	
Sinus (Optimed)	5, 6, 7, 8, 9	20, 30, 40	9–6 10–7	40	Open	N
Vivexx (Bard)	5, 6, 7, 8, 9, 10, 11, 12	20, 30, 40	8–6 10–7 12–8	30, 40 30, 40 30, 40	Open	N
Zilver (Cook)	6, 7, 8, 9, 10	20, 30, 40, 60, 80	NA	NA	Open	N

Nextstent (Boston Scientific)	4, 5, 6, 7, 8, 9, 10	30	9–4	30	Closed	N
Nitrinol (Medinol)	5, 6, 7, 8	21, 30, 44	8–6 10–7	30, 44 30, 44	Closed	N
Wallstent (Boston–Scientific)	6, 7, 8, 9, 10	20, 30, 40	NA	NA	Closed	SS
XACT (Abott)	7, 8, 9, 10	20, 30, 40	8–6 9–7 10–8	30, 40 30, 40 30, 40	Closed	N

N, nitinol; NA, not applicable; SS, stainless steel.

Adapted from Henry et al. Carotid angioplasty and stenting under protection: techniques, indications, results, and limitations. *Textbook of peripheral vascular interventions*, 2nd ed. London: Informa Healthcare;2008: 300–335, with permission of the publisher.

Self-expandable stents notably do not appose the arterial wall as well as balloon-expandable stents; therefore, 1 mm of diameter is typically added during stent selection to accommodate for this difference.[4] Self-expandable stents can be difficult to position because of forward slippage during deployment; thus, cautious backward tension prior to deployment will help avert geographic miss. Most operators in our lab choose to post-dilate with a short 5 or 6 mm balloon (balloon size equal to the diameter of the internal carotid artery) at nominal pressure. After stent placement, the embolic protection device and wire are removed as a unit. Final angiography of the ipsilateral common and internal carotid arteries, as well as of the anterior cerebral circulation, should be performed to exclude embolization or vessel trauma.

Conclusion

- Carotid stenting is a safe and effective alternative to carotid endarterectomy in patients with severe carotid artery occlusive disease and high surgical risk.[6]
- A thoughtful approach to patient selection and meticulous attention to procedural detail will pay dividends in patient outcomes.

Practical Pearls

- Meticulous attention to "de-airing" the system is critical during carotid or intracranial interventions/angiography.
- Always allow back bleeding through the Tuhoy-Borst® adapter after each equipment exchange.
- Limiting EPD dwell time to 30 minutes may help prevent device-related complications.
- Predilation of the lesion is typically necessary to allow passage of the stent across the lesion.
- A buddy wire technique or use of the Emboshield® cerebral protection system may be useful in a tortuous or angulated carotid.
- Right brachial access with an internal mammary artery guide may facilitate carotid intervention in a type III aortic arch.
- Extreme caution in positioning self-expanding stents will dissuade geographic miss.
- Appropriate guide selection is paramount in difficult lesions.
- Assistance from a more experienced operator is invaluable.

References

1. Bates ER, Babb JD, Casey DE, Jr., et al. ACCF/SCAI/SVMB/SIR/ASITN 2007 Clinical Expert Consensus Document on carotid stenting. *Vasc Med.* 2007;12(1):35-83.
2. Bush RL, Lin PH, Mureebe L, Zhou W, Peden EK, Lumsden AB. Routine bivalirudin use in percutaneous carotid interventions. *J Endovasc Ther.* 2005;12(4):521-522.

3. Kapadia SR, Bajzer CT, Ziada KM, et al. Initial experience of platelet glycoprotein IIb/IIIa inhibition with abciximab during carotid stenting: a safe and effective adjunctive therapy. *Stroke.* 2001;32(10):2328-2332.

4. Casserly IP and Yadav JS Carotid intervention. In: Yadav J, Casserly I, Sachar R, eds. *Manual of peripheral vascular intervention.* Philadelphia: Lippincott Williams & Wilkins; 2005:83-109.

5. Mukherjee D and Yadav JS. Carotid angioplasty and stenting under protection: techniques, indications, results, and limitations. In: Henry M, Polydorou A, Henry I, et al., eds. *Textbook of peripheral vascular interventions.* London: Informa Healthcare; 2003:333-341.

6. Helton TJ, Bavry AA, Rajagopal V, et al. The optimal treatment of carotid atherosclerosis: a 2008 update and literature review. *Postgrad Med.* 2008;120(3):103-112.

Chapter 11c

Lower Extremity Arterial Interventions

Saif Anwaruddin and R. David Anderson

Lower extremity peripheral arterial disease (PAD) can be symptomatic or asymptomatic in nature. That atherosclerosis is the pathological culprit is perhaps no surprise, given that PAD shares several risk factors with coronary artery disease, including age, male gender, hypertension, dyslipidemia, cigarette smoking, and diabetes mellitus. Symptomatic lower extremity PAD most often presents as intermittent claudication. It can manifest as rest pain—a poor prognostic sign—which can advance to ulceration and limb loss. A patient's symptoms depend on the anatomic level of obstruction. The prevalence of PAD increases with age, from 8%–10% of those between the ages of 60 and 69 to more than 18% in patients over the age of 70.

Lower extremity atherosclerotic disease can involve any anatomic segment from the iliac arteries proximally to the infrapopliteal vessels distally. Claudication can be graded by the Fontaine or Rutherford classifications (Table 11c.1a).[1] The Transatlantic Inter-Society Consensus (TASC II) classification grades disease on the basis of lesion characteristics (Table 11c.1b).[2] The approach to intervention, including access and equipment selection, will depend on the extent and location of disease.

Patient Management

Prior to any intervention, the treatment of diabetes, hypertension, and dyslipidemia should be maximized. Patients should be on an antiplatelet therapy, such as aspirin. Following percutaneous intervention, clopidogrel is recommended for at least 4 weeks. At the time of the procedure, after access is obtained and a sheath is placed, intravenous heparin is administered with a goal activated clotting time (ACT) of greater than 250 seconds. There are emerging data on substituting bivalirudin for heparin and for using adjuvant therapy, such as glycoprotein IIb/IIIa inhibitors, during these procedures.[3,4] As lower extremity interventions can be prolonged, it is important to recheck the ACT periodically and treat accordingly.

Table 11c.1a Classification of symptomatic peripheral arterial disease (PAD)

Fontaine classification of PAD

Stage I	Asymptomatic
Stage IIa	Mild claudication (>200 M)
Stage IIb	Moderate to severe claudication (≤200 m)
Stage III	Ischemic rest pain
Stage IV	Tissue loss or ulceration

Rutherford Classification of PAD

Grade 0	Category 0	Asymptomatic
Grade 1	Category 1	Mild claudication
Grade 1	Category 2	Moderate claudication
Grade 1	Category 3	Severe claudication
Grade 2	Category 4	Ischemic rest pain
Grade 3	Category 5	Mild tissue ulceration
Grade 3	Category 6	Tissue loss/gangrene

Table 11c.1b TASC II Classification of femoral popliteal lesions

TASC A

- Single stenosis ≤10 cm in length
- Single occlusion ≤5 cm in length

Endovascular therapy is the treatment of choice.

TASC B

- Multiple lesions each ≤5 cm (stenoses or occlusions)
- Single stenosis or occlusion ≤15 cm not involving the infrageniculate popliteal artery
- Single or multiple lesions in the absence of a continuous tibial vessel to improve inflow for a distal bypass
- Heavily calcified occlusion ≤5 cm long
- Single popliteal stenosis

Endovascular therapy is the preferred treatment.

TASC C

- Multiple stenoses or occlusions totaling >15 cm in length, with or without heavy calcification
- Recurrent stenoses or occlusions that need treatment after two endovascular interventions

Surgery is the preferred treatment for good risk patients.

TASC D

- Chronic total occlusion of the common femoral artery or SFA >20 cm in length involving the popliteal artery
- Chronic total occlusion of popliteal artery and proximal trifurcation vessels

Surgery is the treatment of choice.

Iliac Disease

Arterial access for iliac intervention depends on the location of the lesion. Reviewing prior angiograms and/or computed tomography (CT) scans can be helpful in deciding upon a strategy. Proximal common iliac artery disease can be treated from an ipsilateral retrograde approach, whereas distal external iliac disease should be treated using contralateral access and an antegrade approach. Both ipsilateral and contralateral access may be required for chronic total occlusions or for treatment of aortoiliac bifurcation disease. If unable to secure access via the femoral artery, brachial arterial access may be considered.

Treatment of iliac artery disease initially consists of balloon angioplasty. Provisional stenting is reserved for dissections, long or multifocal lesions, chronic total occlusions, extensive calcification, poor runoff, or restenotic disease. Successful balloon angioplasty results in a narrowing of less than 30% or in a translesional gradient of less than 5 mm Hg. Long term patency rates of greater than 70% at 5 years have been reported.[5,6]

For contralateral access, begin by placement of a 5 Fr sheath. A 5 Fr Judkins right or an internal mammary artery diagnostic catheter can be used to obtain access to the contralateral iliac artery. Once achieved, advance a 0.035-inch wire (Wholey or angled Glide Wire) into the contralateral common femoral artery (CFA) or superficial femoral artery (SFA). These guidewires can be exchanged, if needed, for a more supportive wire (Amplatz or Amplatz Superstiff) to allow deployment of a cross-over sheath, such as a Balkin or Destination, into the contralateral iliac artery. This technique can also be used to treat disease distal to the iliac arteries.

Good long-term patency of iliac arteries has been documented with balloon angioplasty alone; however, suboptimal balloon angioplasty of an iliac lesion will require treatment with stent implantation. Characteristics such as lesion location, access site, sheath size, side-branch patency, and proximity to the CFA affect stent choice. Common iliac disease extending into the distal aorta or with heavy calcification is typically treated with balloon-expandable stents. These stents are sized in a 1:1 stent-to-artery fashion. Given their physical characteristics and the tortuosity of the mid-iliac vessels, balloon-expandable stents are generally avoided in mid-common and external iliac arteries. Self-expanding stents are more commonly used in these locations. Disease involving or in proximity to the CFA should be treated without stenting if at all possible. If required due to suboptimal results, self-expanding nitinol stents are preferred here owing to their flexibility. They may occasionally be used in tortuous vessels or in cases of contralateral access, where tracking larger balloon-expandable stents may be challenging. When using self-expanding stents, it is preferable to upsize stent diameter by 1 mm for any given vessel size. Postdilatation is more often necessary with self-expanding stents than with balloon-expandable stents. It is important to note when deploying self-expanding stents that exact placement of the stent may be challenging given the need to unsheath these devices during deployment (Fig. 11c.1a,b).

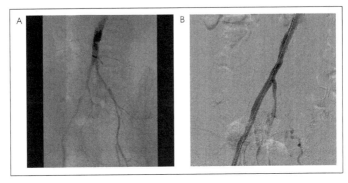

Figure 11c.1 Iliac artery disease. (A) Aortoiliac angiogram demonstrating severe disease of the right external iliac artery. Previous stent noted in the right common iliac artery. (B) Right external iliac artery following balloon angioplasty and stenting. Previous stent is noted in the right common iliac artery.

Femoropopliteal Disease

For CFA disease, consideration must be given to the choice between percutaneous and surgical treatment. If percutaneous therapy is warranted, access should be obtained via the contralateral side using the cross-over technique described earlier. Ideally, one should avoid stenting the CFA. This can lead to a high rate of stent fracture or restenosis, due to a high degree of flexion and extension of the hip joint. This also limits future percutaneous and surgical access. Balloon angioplasty alone or atherectomy devices to debulk lesions (see Table 11c.2) in the CFA are the preferred strategies to avoid the use of a stent. If stenting is necessary, consideration should be given to self-expanding nitinol stents (Fig. 11c.2).

To properly treat symptomatic disease of the SFA, it is important to understand the anatomy of the vessel as it courses below the femoral head, down into the adductor canal, and toward the popliteal fossa. Lateral and posterior to the SFA, the profunda femoral artery branches off the CFA. The importance of the profunda branch is in often providing collateral supply to a proximally occluded SFA. Compromise of the profunda femoral artery should be avoided at all costs.[7]

Arterial access for treating SFA disease is obtained by contralateral access and crossing over, as described earlier, specifically favoring a 7 Fr system. Other options include ipsilateral access using an antegrade approach, an upper extremity approach as noted previously, or less commonly, a retrograde approach from the popliteal, dorsalis pedis, or posterior tibial arteries. The ipsilateral antegrade approach may be used when the aortoiliac anatomy precludes a contralateral cross-over approach (Fig. 11c.3). Once access is obtained, intravenous heparin should be administered, as previously described.

Table 11c.2 Atherectomy devices

- Rotational Atherectomy (Boston Scientific)
- Silverhawk Atherectomy (Fox Hollow Technologies/eV3)
- Diamondback Orbital Atherectomy (Cardiovascular Systems Inc.)
- Jetstream G2 Atherectomy (Pathway Medical Technologies)
- Peripheral Atherectomy Catheter – PAC (Arrow International)
- Laser Atherectomy (Spectranetics)

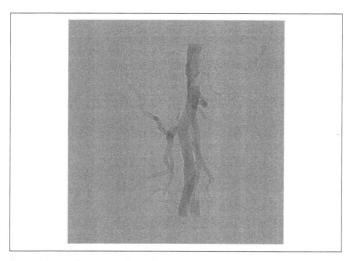

Figure 11c.2 Right common femoral artery stenosis. In this case, an atherectomy device was used to treat the lesion.

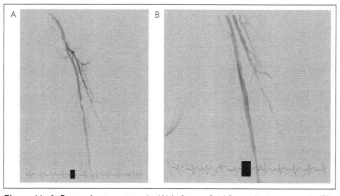

Figure 11c.3 Femoral artery stenosis. (A) Left superficial femoral artery stenosis. (B) Left superficial femoral artery lesion treated with balloon angioplasty and a 7 × 40 mm self-expanding stent (Glide Wire still in place).

Guidewire placement in the SFA can be accomplished using a 0.035-inch Wholey wire or a hydrophilic Glide Wire. A Glide catheter can be used to provide support. Balloon angioplasty is carefully performed to avoid arterial dissection. Stent revascularization of the SFA with self-expanding nitinol stents has been considered to be superior to balloon angioplasty, but a recent meta-analysis questions this strategy.[8] Stenting should be reserved for lesions longer than 5 cm, dissection, multiple stenoses, heavy calcification, and treatment of restenosis.[9] The primary concern with the use of stents in the SFA is stent fracture. The use of atherectomy devices is also an option that can be considered when trying to avoid stent placement, and several devices are available for use (Table 11c.3).

Infrapopliteal Disease

Disease below the level of the popliteal artery requires a well thought-out approach prior to intervention. Treatment of these vessels is usually reserved for limb ischemia, as patency rates are lower.[10] Consideration should be given to revascularization of the branches that supply the majority of the distal

Table 11c.3 Complications of lower extremity interventions

Complication	Initial Evaluation and Management	Treatment	Comments
Dissection	Assess if dissection is flow-limiting; if not, then nothing further may be necessary.	If flow-limiting, prolonged balloon inflation + stenting	Type of stent to be used should be determined by anatomic level of dissection.
Perforation	Discontinue/reverse anticoagulation, fluid resuscitation (if necessary), prolonged balloon inflation.	Covered stent required if bleeding does not stop after initial management	Watch closely for signs of compartment syndrome, necessitating surgical intervention.
Thrombosis	Ensure no underlying dissection as a cause.	Mechanical thrombectomy, thrombolysis	
Vasospasm	Ensure no underlying dissection as a cause.	Intra-arterial nitrates and calcium channel blockers	More common with infrapopliteal interventions
Distal embolization	No-reflow or vessel cutoff during procedure	Pharmacological vs. mechanical aspiration depending on size	In lesions with heavy thrombus burden consider use of embolic protection device. For large embolization, surgical intervention may be required.

extremity. Approach can be a contralateral cross-over approach or an ipsilateral antegrade approach for more distal infrapopliteal disease. Typically, for infrapopliteal interventions, a 0.014-inch wire is used to cross the lesion, and coronary balloons are used for dilation. Stenting at this level should be reserved for complications, such as dissections or residual stenosis. There are small studies demonstrating the efficacy of drug-eluting coronary stents over bare metal stents for bail-out stenting.[11]

Complications

Please see Table 11c.3 for special issues related to managing complications of lower extremity interventions.

Conclusion

- Interventions performed on symptomatic lower extremity arterial disease require careful planning regarding decisions about access site and equipment.
- The level of obstructive disease, in addition to other lesion characteristics, will help to determine the percutaneous strategy used for an individual patient.

Practical Pearls

- Planning ahead, with an understanding of both the symptom and lesion classification, as well as your anticipated interventional strategy, will minimize procedural difficulties.
- Always check equipment stock pre-procedure to be certain that balloons, stents, wires, catheters, and sheaths of the appropriate diameters and lengths are available.
- When performing aortoiliac interventions, avoid antithrombotic agents that cannot be reversed in the event of a misadventure such as perforation.
- Be certain to have on hand equipment needed for bail-outs, such as a large (12–14 mm) balloon for distal aortic occlusion and covered stents.
- Always maintain adequate anticoagulation and confirm activated clotting time (ACT goal >250 sec) if using heparin. Repeat check every 30–45 minutes for prolonged procedures and re-dose as necessary.
- There is nothing wrong with an adequate balloon result.

References

1. Management of peripheral arterial disease (PAD). Transatlantic Inter-Society Consensus (TASC). *Eur J Vasc Endovasc Surg.* 2000;19 (Suppl A):Si-xxviii, S1-250.
2. Norgren L, Hiatt WR, Dormandy JA, Nehler MR, Harris KA, Fowkes FG; TASC II Working Group. Inter-Society consensus for the management of peripheral arterial disease (TASC II). *J Vasc Surg.* 2007;45 (Suppl S):S5-67.

3. Allie DE, Hall P, Shammas NW, et al. The Angiomax Peripheral Procedure Registry of Vascular Events trial (APPROVE): in-hospital and 30-day results. *J Invasive Cardiol.* 2004;16:651-656.

4. Shammas NW. Complications in peripheral vascular interventions: emerging role of direct thrombin inhibitors. *J Vasc Interv Radiol.* 2005;16:165-171.

5. Calabrese E. Infrapopliteal arterial diseases: angioplasty and stenting. In: Heuser RR, Henry M, eds. *Textbook of peripheral vascular interventions,* 2nd ed. London: Informa HealthCare, 2008:633-638.

6. Roffi M, Biamino G. Aortic, iliac, and common femoral intervention. In: Casserly IP, Sachar R, Yadav JS, eds. *Manual of peripheral vascular intervention.* Philadelphia: Lippincott Williams & Wilkins, 2005:214-228.

7. Goldstein JA, Casserly IP, Rocha-Singh K. Endovascular therapy for superficial femoral arterial disease. In: Casserly IP, Sachar R, Yadav JS, eds. *Manual of peripheral vascular intervention.* Philadelphia: Lippincott Williams & Wilkins, 2005::229-251.

8. Kasapis C, Henke PK, Chetcuti SJ, et al. Routine stent implantation vs. percutaneous transluminal angioplasty in femoropopliteal artery disease: a meta-analysis of randomized controlled trials. *Eur Heart J.* 2009;30:44-55.

9. Schillinger M, Sabeti S, Loewe C, et al. Balloon angioplasty versus implantation of nitinol stents in the superficial femoral artery. *N Engl J Med.* 2006:354: 1879-1888.

10. Hirsch AT, Haskal Ziv J, Hertzer NR, et al. ACC/AHA 2005 Guidelines for the management of patients with peripheral arterial disease (lower extremity, renal, mesenteric, and abdominal aortic): a collaborative report from the American Association for Vascular Surgery/Society for Vascular Surgery, Society for Cardiovascular Angiography and Interventions, Society for Vascular Medicine and Biology, Society of Interventional Radiology, and the ACC/AHA Task Force on Practice Guidelines (Writing Committee to Develop Guidelines for the Management of Patients with Peripheral Arterial Disease). *J Am Coll Cardiol.* 2006;47:e1-e192.

11. Siablis D, Karnabatidis D, Katsanos K, et al. Sirolimus-eluting versus bare stents after suboptimal infrapopliteal angioplasty for critical limb ischemia: enduring 1-year angiographic and clinical benefit. *J Endovasc Ther.* 2007;14:241-250.

Chapter 12

Structural Heart Disease

Chapter 12a

Atrial Septal Defect/Patent Foramen Ovale Closure

Ryan D'Souza and Bernhard Meier

An atrial septal defect (ASD) is a lesion in the interatrial septum. It is a common form of congenital heart disease and accounts for 10% of all congenital heart diseases.[1] There are three types of ASDs (ostium secundum, ostium primum, and sinus venosus), each with different anatomical or clinical features and therapeutic options. Although surgical therapy remains the standard treatment for the latter two defects, percutaneous closure of secundum ASD is a safe alternative,[2] and the therapy of choice for ASDs up to 30 mm in size.

The foramen ovale is a valve-like opening of the interatrial septum during intrauterine life. The interatrial septum is made from two overlapping embryological structures, the left-sided partially fibrous septum primum and the right-sided muscular septum secundum. These grow from the periphery to the center, leaving a central opening, called the foramen ovale, with the septum primum serving as a one-way slit valve for physiological right-to-left shunt during in utero development. The blood flow from the umbilical vein entering the right atrium through the inferior vena cava bypasses the collapsed lungs, keeping the foramen ovale open until after birth. The postnatal enhancement of the pulmonary circulation leads to a decrease of the right atrial pressure to a level below left atrial pressure. This results in functional closure of the foramen ovale by apposition of the septum primum against the septum secundum. In the ensuing months, the caudal portion of the septum primum on the left side and the cranial portion of the septum secundum on the right side fuse permanently. Autopsy studies have shown that the foramen ovale remains patent in about one-quarter of the general population.[3]

Atrial septal aneurysm (ASA) is the term used to describe a congenital abnormality of the interatrial septum characterized by a redundant, muscular membrane in the region of the fossa ovalis. It is one of the reasons why the patent foramen ovale (PFO) persists. The prevalence of ASA in the general population was about 1% in autopsy series,[4–6] and 2.2% in a population-based transesophageal echocardiographic (TEE) study.[7] An ASA is associated with a PFO in 50%–85% of cases, which constitutes a three- to five-fold increased risk for recurrent embolic events compared to patients with PFO alone.[8]

Indications for Atrial Septal Defect/Patent Foramen Ovale Closure

Secundum ASDs associated with echocardiographic findings of right atrial and ventricular volume overload or catheterization findings of a pulmonary-to-systemic flow ratio (Qp:Qs) of greater than 1.5:1 need to be closed for hemodynamic reasons. Atrial septal defects may cause paradoxical embolism, which is another reason to close them. Small ASDs are easier to close, to compensate for the less compelling indications.

Patent foramen ovales are increasingly recognized as potential mediators of several disease manifestations, in addition to paradoxical embolism, which is the most important[9–15] (Table 12a.1). At present, the most restrictive indications for PFO closure are applied in the United States, with the sole accepted U.S. Food and Drug Administration (FDA) indication being failed medical treatment for secondary stroke prevention.

Closure Devices

Various devices are available for percutaneous ASD closure (Fig. 12a.1). The only two FDA-approved devices for percutaneous ASD closure are the Amplatzer Septal Occluder (ASO) (AGA Medical Corporation, Plymouth, MN) and the Gore Helix device (WL Gore & Associates, Flag Staff, AZ). We routinely use the ASO device (Table 12a.2).

Anatomic and physiological differences between PFO and ASD led to development of devices specifically meant for percutaneous PFO closure (Fig. 12a.2). We predominantly use the Amplatzer PFO Occluder (APFO) (AGA Medical Corporation, Plymouth, MN) (Table 12a.3). Using the current generation of devices, complete closure rates of more than 90% of cases can be expected.[16]

Technique

Every patient should undergo TEE (Figs. 12a.3 and 12a.4) prior to intervention for initial diagnosis of the defect and detailed evaluation of the anatomy. The actual percutaneous ASD/PFO closures can be performed under local anesthesia, using only fluoroscopic guidance. Although most centers perform percutaneous ASD/PFO closure under TEE[17] or intracardiac echocardiography (ICE)[18] guidance, we do not advocate this for various reasons[19] (Tables 12a.4, 12a.5). Complications of ASD/PFO closure[20] (Table 12a.6) depend on experience of the operator, type of device used, and characteristics of the defect.

The patient is adequately anticoagulated with unfractionated heparin. A venous access is gained via the right femoral vein.

Table 12a.1 Conditions associated with patent foramen ovale

- Paradoxical embolism[9]
- Orthostatic desaturation in the setting of the rare platypnea–orthodeoxia syndrome[10]
- Refractory hypoxemia due to right to left shunt in patients with right ventricular infarction[11] or severe pulmonary disease
- Neurological decompression illness in divers[12]
- Migraine with aura[13]
- Transient global amnesia
- Obstructive sleep apnoea[14]
- High-altitude pulmonary edema[15]

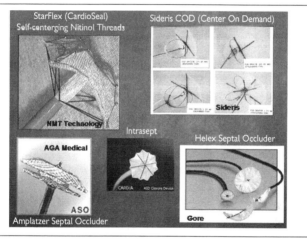

Figure 12a.1 Selected percutaneous atrial septal defect closure devices. The manufacturers are imprinted on the pictures.

Table 12a.2 Specific characteristics of Amplatzer Septal Occluder device

- Self-expanding and self-retaining double-disk device
- Manufactured from 0.005-inch nitinol wire
- Two expandable round disks with a 4-mm-long connecting waist
- Polymer fabric patch is sewn into the left and right atrial disks and the connecting waist to enhance tissue ingrowth.
- Fully recoverable and repositionable when attached to the delivery cable
- Available in sizes ranging from 4 to 42 mm
- Size is indicated by the diameter of the waist.
- Left disk is larger than the right disk.
- Delivery system consists of pusher cable, loader, and delivery sheath (6–13 Fr)

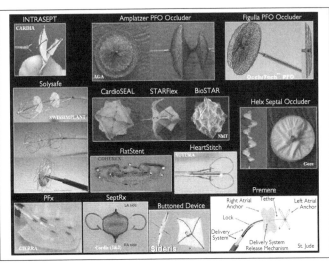

Figure 12a.2 Selected percutaneous patent foramen ovale closure devices. The manufacturers are imprinted on the pictures.

Table 12a.3 Specific characteristics of Amplatzer Patent Foramen Ovale Occluder device

- Manufactured from 0.005-inch nitinol wire
- Polyester fabric patch sewn into both disks
- Left atrial disk is smaller than or equal to the right disk.
- Thin flexible waist connects the two retention disks.
- Available in 18, 25, 30, 35, and 40 mm sizes
- Dominant right atrial disk measures 25 and 35 mm.
- Nondominant left atrial disk measures 18 and 22 mm, respectively.
- Fits through 8 or 9 Fr delivery sheath

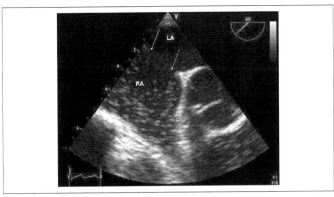

Figure 12a.3 Transesophageal echocardiography showing an atrial septal defect **between the arrows,** functionally proved by a washout zone in the adjacent right atrium (RA) during a bubble test. LA, left atrium.

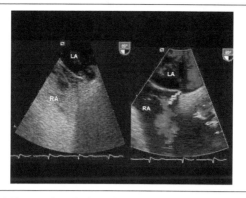

Figure 12a.4 Transesophageal echocardiography proving a patent foramen ovale by passage of aerated saline appearing as bubbles (*left*) and as a Doppler shunt (*right*) through a patent foramen ovale after a Valsalva maneuver. Patency of the foramen ovale can be semiquantitatively assessed by counting the number of bubbles in the left atrium on a still frame: small shunt (0–5 bubbles), moderate shunt (6–20 bubbles), large shunt (>20 bubbles). LA, left atrium; RA, right atrium.

Table 12a.4 Disadvantages of intraprocedural transesophageal echocardiography

- Prolongs procedure time
- Poorly tolerated by supine patients
- Risks associated with sedation/general anesthesia
- Intubation may be required to prevent bronchial aspiration

Table 12a.5 Disadvantages of intraprocedural intracardiac echocardiography

- Prolongs procedure time
- Costly
- Increases the invasive risk (second access, rigid, unguided intravenous catheter)

Atrial Septal Defect Closure

The ASD is crossed under fluoroscopic guidance in the anteroposterior (AP) view, using a J-tip standard length 0.035-inch guidewire, and, if required, the help of a 6 Fr multipurpose catheter or similar device (Fig. 12a.5). Balloon sizing of the ASD using an AGA Amplatzer sizing balloon is done in the projection that best separates the two distal closely spaced markers (Fig. 12a.6). This confirms that the balloon is being viewed perpendicularly and is not foreshortened. The distance between the leading edge of the proximal marker and the leading edge of the first distal marker is 15 mm for reference. The balloon is inflated with diluted contrast medium until a waist is seen on both sides. It should not be overinflated, to avoid tearing the septum (Fig. 12a.7). If echocardiography

Table 12a.6 Complications or failures of percutaneous atrial septal defect/patent foramen ovale (ASD/PFO) closure

Thrombus formation on device	No risk acutely if procedural time short and patient adequately anticoagulated. Mostly seen with Cardio SEAL device (NMT Medical, Boston, MA) in initial months.
Tear of atrial septum	Avoid overstretching sizing balloon.
Device migration	Infrequent and mostly not life-threatening. Can be retrieved in the catheterization laboratory or operating room.
Cardiac perforation	Incidence is 0.1%.[20]
Residual shunts	Mostly small and hemodynamically insignificant. Devices may act as clot filters. If large, can be treated by a repeat procedure.
Complications related to vascular access such as hematomas, arteriovenous fistulae, and false aneurysms	Avoid an arterial puncture.

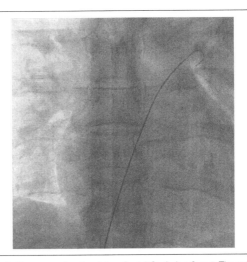

Figure 12a.5 Placement of an Amplatzer Septal Occluder. Step 1: The atrial septal defect is crossed under fluoroscopic guidance in the anteroposterior view, using a guidewire or a curved catheter.

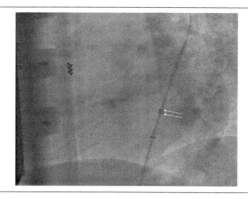

Figure 12a.6 Placement of an Amplatzer Septal Occluder. Step 2: Balloon-sizing of the atrial septal defect using AGA Amplatzer sizing balloon in the projection which best separates the distal two closely spaced markers on the balloon (*arrows*).

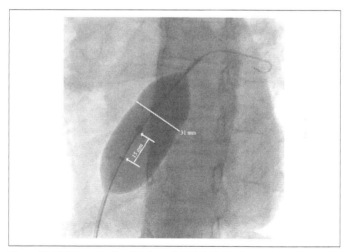

Figure 12a.7 Placement of an Amplatzer Septal Occluder. Step 3: The diameter of the waist of the sizing balloon indicates the stretched diameter of the defect.

is used, the balloon is inflated until a Doppler shunt across the defect ceases (stop-flow technique). An Amplatzer Septal Occluder device 20%–50% larger than the balloon stretched diameter of the ASD is selected. More oversizing is needed in case it is difficult to stabilize the inflated balloon, which indicates flimsy rims. The device is prepared before introducing the sheath to reduce the indwelling time of the sheath. The device is screwed onto the pusher cable, loosened by unscrewing by a fraction of a turn, and drawn into the loader sheath under water to avoid air entrapment. The tip of the device is kept peeking out of the loader by a few millimeters to avoid air entrapment while connecting it to the sheath (Fig. 12a.8).

The delivery sheath, along with its dilator, is advanced over the guidewire until the tip of the sheath is at the entrance of a pulmonary vein or the left atrial appendage (Fig. 12a.9). To prevent air from being sucked in while removing the dilator, the delivery sheath at its proximal exit is kept lateral to the patient's thigh, below the level of the heart. Further, as the dilator of the sheath is pulled back, the guidewire is kept in the left atrium. This prevents wedging of the end hole of the delivery sheath against the wall and allows blood to follow the receding dilator, filling the void and preventing inadvertent aspiration of air. After the dilator and guidewire are removed, the loader is connected to the delivery sheath and the device is advanced under fluoroscopic guidance in the AP view to the left atrium, by advancing the pusher cable. Before exiting the sheath, ascertain that the device is correctly screwed onto the pusher cable (Fig. 12a.10). The left atrial disk, along with the connector and a small part of the right disk, is then deployed in the left atrium, under fluoroscopy in the left

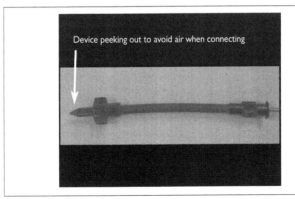

Device peeking out to avoid air when connecting

Figure 12a.8 Placement of an Amplatzer Septal Occluder. Step 4: Device within the loader ready for connection with the delivery sheath.

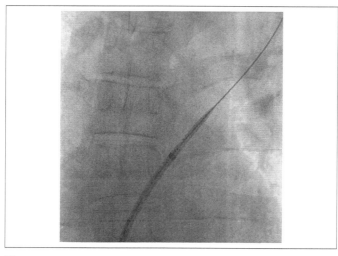

Figure 12a.9 Placement of an Amplatzer Septal Occluder. Step 5: The delivery sheath along with the dilator is introduced on the guidewire into the left atrium.

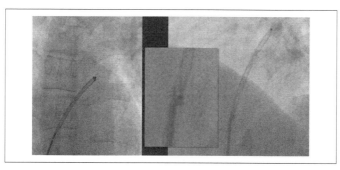

Figure 12a.10 Placement of an Amplatzer Septal Occluder. Step 6: Ascertain that the device is properly screwed onto the pusher cable before exiting from the sheath (*left*). The two images on the right show that the device was unscrewed from the pusher cable.

anterior oblique (LAO) projection (Fig. 12a.11). Deployment of a small part of the right atrial disk ensures that the device is pulled through the center of the defect, thereby preventing prolapse of the left upper disk before the right disk is positioned. The entire system is withdrawn until the left atrial disk leans against the left atrial side of the atrial septum. The tip of the sheath is then further withdrawn (Fig. 12a.12), following which the right atrial component of the device is fully expanded in the right atrium (Fig. 12a.13). Gentle wiggling

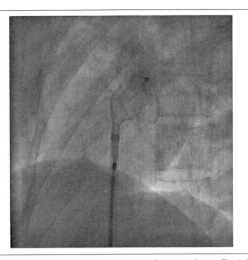

Figure 12a.11 Placement of an Amplatzer Septal Occluder. Step 7: The left atrial disk, the connector, and a small part of the right disk are deployed deep within the left atrium.

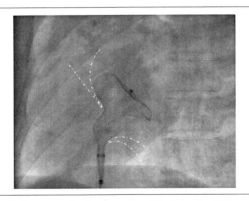

Figure 12a.12 Placement of an Amplatzer Septal Occluder. Step 8: The entire system is withdrawn until the left atrial disk abuts against the cranial left atrial side of the septum. The caudal part of the right disk is not yet in the right atrium in this picture. The septum is indicated by the dashed lines.

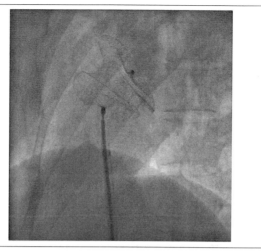

Figure 12a.13 Placement of an Amplatzer Septal Occluder. Step 9: The right atrial disk is now fully in the right atrium.

is performed to ensure device placement in a stable position. Potential air is purged from the sheath, and a right atrial contrast angiogram is done through a Y connector plugged onto the delivery sheath, to delineate the right atrial septum (Fig. 12a.14). Following the contrast medium through to the levophase, the left atrial septal border can also be assessed. If echocardiography is used, the passage of the septum between the disks is checked. The delivery wire is then unscrewed and the device released. The delivery sheath is used for a final contrast medium injection (Fig. 12a.15), which is again followed to the levophase to delineate the left atrial contour and disk placement.

Patent Foramen Ovale Closure

After gaining venous access through the right femoral vein, the PFO is crossed under fluoroscopic guidance in the AP view using a J-tip standard length 0.035-inch guidewire alone, or, if required, with the help of a 6 Fr multipurpose or similarly shaped catheter. Occasionally (small PFO), the J-tip of the wire has to be straightened before it will cross the defect. Balloon sizing is not used, as the maximal opening of the flaplike PFO is not crucial for successful closure (in addition, there is a finite risk of the measuring balloon tearing the thin septum primum). A 25 mm Amplatzer PFO Occluder is routinely selected for most cases, except for tiny PFOs with extremely low mobility (18 mm), or very long tunnels and large PFOs with flimsy rims, in which large occluders are used in about 5% of cases. In contrast to ASD closure, only the left atrial disk is deployed into the left atrium (Fig. 12a.16) before the device and sheath

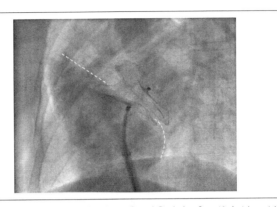

Figure 12a.14 Placement of an Amplatzer Septal Occluder. Step 10: A right atrial contrast angiogram delineates the atrial septum (*dashed lines*). The device should be visualized in perfect profile without any disk overlap. The device is then released.

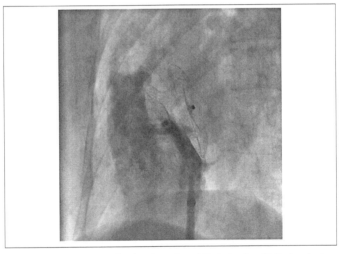

Figure 12a.15 Placement of an Amplatzer Septal Occluder. Step 11: Final contrast angiogram after the device is released.

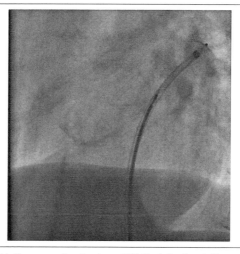

Figure 12a.16 Placement of an Amplatzer PFO Occluder. Step 1: The patent foramen ovale is crossed, and the delivery sheath introduced as illustrated in Figures 12a.5 and 12a.9. The left disk of the Amplatzer PFO Occluder is released deep in the left atrium.

are gently pulled back together as a unit against the atrial septum under fluoroscopy in a LAO projection (Fig. 12a.17). The right atrial disk is deployed by maintaining tension on the pusher cable while further withdrawing the delivery sheath (Fig. 12a.18). The Pacman sign,[21] refers to the position of the device, which should be ascertained on fluoroscopy, or echocardiography if used, before release (Fig. 12a.19). After verification of correct position and stability of the device, a right atrial contrast angiogram is done to delineate the atrial septum (Fig. 12a.20). Ideally, the levophase is also filmed. The device is wiggled to check for stability and then released by unscrewing the pusher cable in counterclockwise fashion. A final contrast injection is done and followed until the levophase to delineate the left atrial contour and disk placement (Fig. 12a.21).

After the procedure, the sheath is removed, and hemostasis is achieved by manual compression of the venous puncture, which can easily be accomplished by the patient himself. One dose of antibiotic is administered in the catheterization laboratory, followed by one or two more doses over the next 12 hours, although the use of antibiotics is not supported by evidence. Acetylsalicylic acid (ASA, aspirin) (100 mg once daily) for 5 months and clopidogrel (75 mg once daily) for 1 month is prescribed for antithrombotic protection.

A transthoracic contrast echocardiogram is done before discharge to document correct and stable position of the device. A contrast TEE is repeated after 6 months, ideally 1 month after stopping therapy to assess the freedom of

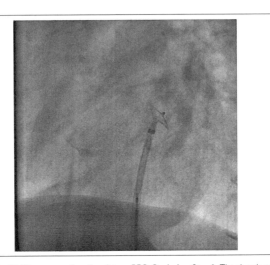

Figure 12a.17 Placement of an Amplatzer PFO Occluder. Step 2: The sheath and device are pulled back as a unit against the septum.

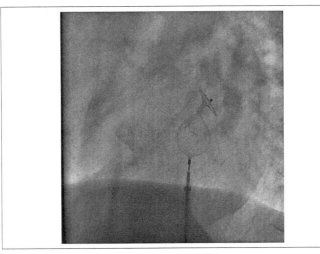

Figure 12a.18 Placement of Amplatzer PFO Occluder. Step 3: The right atrial disk is unfolded in the right atrium.

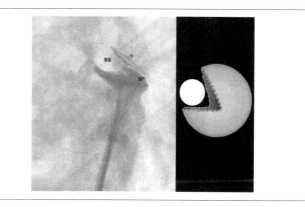

Figure 12a.19 Placement of an Amplatzer PFO Occluder. Step 4: The Pacman sign is a reliable marker for correct device position prior to release. The device appears to bite into the thick, muscular septum secundum (ss) cranially (*left*), while the disks are less separated by the paper thin septum primum (sp) caudally (*right*). This feature is reminiscent of the vintage arcade game figure Pacman© about to gobble up a dot (on the right).

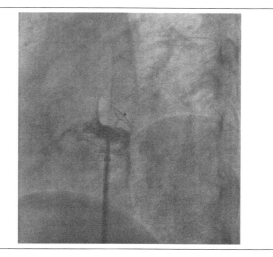

Figure 12a.20 Placement of an Amplatzer PFO Occluder. Step 5: A right atrial contrast angiogram delineates the atrial septum and correct position of device before release.

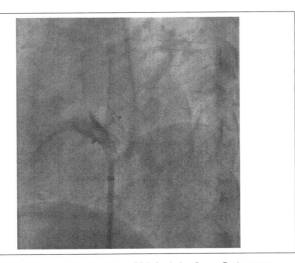

Figure 12a.21 Placement of an Amplatzer PFO Occluder. Step 6: Final contrast angiogram after the device is released.

thrombus without platelet inhibitors. Small residual shunts may be left as the device filters out particles. In case of a significant residual shunt, implantation of a second device is recommended, which results in complete closure in about 90% of such cases.

Future Developments

Newer devices being investigated for percutaneous ASD or PFO closure are bioabsorbable devices, or device-free techniques (PFO only) to avoid permanent foreign bodies in the heart. However, resorbable devices harbor the risk of recurrent shunts and embolization of fragments.

The CIERRA PFx closure system was a percutaneous system that employed radiofrequency energy to close the PFO by welding the septum primum and septum secundum together, thus avoiding the need for an implantable device. The device was plagued by low feasibility and high residual shunt rates, requiring subsequent device closure. It has been retracted from use. Other developments include similar ideas and transcatheter suture systems.

Conclusion

- Percutaneous ASD closure has been around for almost 35 years, preceding coronary angioplasty.

- Large ASDs need to be closed, and the majority can be closed percutaneously.
- Small ASDs should also be closed, because they harbor the risk of paradoxical embolism and are easy to close percutaneously.
- Percutaneous closure of a PFO has a high success rate at a very low risk.
- Although there is no randomized proof, PFO closure is sure to yield a net clinical benefit, given time.
- Patent foramen ovales can be closed with a variety of devices.
- The Amplatzer Occluder provides optimal ease of use and results.

Practical Pearls

- For percutaneous closure of simple ASDs and PFOs, echocardiographic guidance is not necessary and omitting it shortens the procedure and reduces risk.
- In the absence of echocardiography, assessment of position in a fluoroscopic view perfectly separating the two disks is essential.
- Percutaneous PFO closure can be learned from an expert in five to ten cases.
- The result seen a few months after the procedure is definitive; late closures are extremely rare.
- A PFO may not be alone (one hole each in both edges of the PFO slit, for instance).
- A marked atrial septal aneurysm is a cause for a PFO, renders it more dangerous, and is often associated with one or several small ASDs.
- The eustachian valve is another cause for and risk factor of a PFO.
- The eustachian valve may prevent bubbles injected from the arm to pass through a PFO and therefore can be a reason for missing the diagnosis of the PFO.

References

1. Carlgren LE. The incidence of congenital heart disease in children born in Gothenburg 1941-1950. *Br Heart J.* 1959;21:40-50.

2. Fisher G, Stieh J, Uebing A, et al. Experience with transcatheter closure of secundum atrial septal defects using the Amplatzer septal occluder: a single centre study in 236 consecutive patients. *Heart.* 2003;89:199-204.

3. Hagen PT, Scholz DG, Edwards WD. Incidence and size of patent foramen ovale during the first 10 decades of life: an autopsy study of 965 normal hearts. *Mayo Clin Proc.* 1984;59:17-20.

4. Silver MD, Dorsey JS. Aneurysms of the septum primum in adults. *Arch Pathol Lab*

5. Med. 1978;102:62–65.

6. Hanley PC, Tajik AJ, Hynes JK, et al. Diagnosis and classification of atrial septal aneurysm by two-dimensional echocardiography: report of 80 consecutive cases. *J Am Coll Cardiol.* 1985;6:1370–1382.

7. Pearson AC, Nagelhout D, Castello R, et al. Atrial septal aneurysm and stroke: a transesophageal echocardiographic study. *J Am Coll Cardiol.* 1991;18:1223–1229.

8. Agmon Y, Khandheria BK, Meissner I, et al. Frequency of atrial septal aneurysms in patients with cerebral ischemic events. *Circulation.* 1999;99:1942–1944.

9. Overell JR, Bone I, Lees KR. Interatrial septal abnormalities and stroke: a meta-analysis of case-control studies. *Neurology.* 2000;55:1172–1179.

10. Lechat P, Mas JL, Lascault G, et al. Prevalence of patent foramen ovale in patients with stroke. *N Engl J Med.* 1988;318:1148–1152.

11. Seward JB, Hayes DL, Smith HC, et al. Platypnea-orthodeoxia: clinical profile, diagnostic workup, management, and report of seven cases. *Mayo Clin Proc.* 1984;59:221–231.

12. Silver MT, Lieberman EH, Thibault GE. Refractory hypoxemia in inferior myocardial infarction from right-to-left shunting through a patent foramen ovale: a case report and review of the literature. *Clin Cardiol.* 1994;17:627 630.

13. Germonpre P, Dendale P, Unger P, Balestra C. Patent foramen ovale and decompression sickness in sports divers. *J Appl Physiol.* 1998;84:1622–1626.

14. Schwerzmann M, Nedeltchev K, Lagger F, et al. Prevalence and size of directly detected patent foramen ovale in migraine with aura. *Neurology.* 2005;65: 1415–1418.

15. Agnoletti G, Iserin L, Lafont A, Sidi D, Desnos M. Obstructive sleep apnoea and patent foramen ovale: successful treatment of symptoms by percutaneous foramen ovale closure. *J Interv Cardiol.* 2005;18:393–395.

16. Allemann Y, Hutter D, Lipp E, et al. Patent foramen ovale and high-altitude pulmonary edema. *JAMA.* 2006;296:2954-2958.

17. Wahl A, Krumsdorf U, Meier B, et al. Transcatheter treatment of atrial septal aneurysm associated with patent foramen ovale for prevention of recurrent paradoxical embolism in high-risk patients. *J Am Coll Cardiol.* 2005;45:377–380.

18. Hung J, Landzberg MJ, Jenkins KJ, et al. Closure of patent foramen ovale for paradoxical emboli: intermediate-term. *J Am Coll Cardiol.* 2000;35:1311–1316.

19. Onorato E, Melzi G, Casilli F, et al. Patent foramen ovale with paradoxical embolism: mid-term results of transcatheter closure in 256 patients. *J Interv Cardiol.* 2003;16:43–50.

20. Meier B. Closure of the patent foramen ovale: the end of the sound and vision era approaching. *JACC Cardiovasc Interv.* 2008;1(4):392-394.

21. Amin Z, Hijazi ZM, Bass JL, et al. Erosion of Amplatzer occluder device after closure of secundum atrial defects: review of registry of complications and recommendations to minimize future risk. *Catheter Cardiovasc Interv.* 2004;63:496-502.

22. Meier B. Pacman sign during device closure of the patent foramen ovale. *Catheter Cardiovasc Interv.* 2003;60:221–223.

Chapter 12b

Ethanol Septal Ablation

Srihari S. Naidu

Previously thought a rare disorder, hypertrophic cardiomyopathy (HCM) is present in 1 in 500 of the population. Symptoms may be vague for many years, reaching clinical significance only once heart failure, syncope, angina, palpitations, or sudden cardiac arrest develop.[1] About half of patients do not have left ventricular outflow tract obstruction, whereas 25% have resting obstruction and an additional 25% have obstruction only with provocation.[2] The presence of obstruction has been linked to worse long-term survival and higher symptomatic status.[3]

Medical therapy with negative inotropic agents improves symptoms in one-half of patients.[1] The remainder, roughly 10% of the total HCM population, are a target for invasive therapy. Surgical myectomy has been the gold standard invasive therapy in experienced centers.[4] However, some patients are not candidates due to advanced age, comorbidity, previous cardiac surgery, poor motivation, a strong desire to avoid open heart surgery, or lack of local expertise in the procedure. In 1994, the first ethanol septal ablation procedure was performed, whereby absolute alcohol was used to induce a localized infarction of the basal septum at the point of anterior mitral valve coaptation, thereby reducing outflow tract gradient and consequent mitral regurgitation (MR).[5] Since then, the procedure has been disseminated widely, with outcomes in appropriately selected patients similar to myectomy.[6]

Patient Management

Patient Selection

Patients must meet specific clinical, echocardiographic, and angiographic criteria (Table 12b.1). Since invasive therapy is only warranted for refractory symptoms despite medical therapy, patients must be on optimal medical therapy at the time invasive therapy is considered. Patients who remain in New York Heart Association (NYHA) heart failure Class III/IV or Canadian Cardiovascular Society (CCS) Angina Class III/IV are candidates.[7,8] In rare instances, patients with lower NYHA or CCS Class may be candidates to treat recurrent gradient-related syncope.

Table 12b.1 Indications and contraindications for ethanol septal ablation	
Clinical	*Accepted*: NYHA Class III–IV or CCS Angina Class III–IV refractory to optimal medical therapy
	Reasonable: Recurrent syncope or pre–syncope, refractory paroxysmal atrial fibrillation with clinical decompensation during episodes
	Contraindicated: Symptoms can be reasonably attributed to alternate diagnosis, i.e., severe obesity or other comorbidity
Echocardiographic	*Accepted*: Asymmetric septal hypertrophy >1.3:1, Systolic anterior motion (SAM) of the anterior mitral valve leaflet, outflow tract gradient at basal septal of >30 mm resting and/or >50–60 mm provocable, posteriorly–directed mitral regurgitation
	Reasonable: Midcavitary obstruction, relatively severe septal thickening >2.5 cm
	Contraindicated: Intrinsic pathology of mitral valve apparatus and/or papillary muscles that requires surgical correction, concomitant cardiac disease that requires surgery (i.e., aortic stenosis), severe septal thickening >3.0 cm
Angiographic	*Accepted*: Septal perforator >1.5 mm in diameter that serves the target myocardium, as determined by intra–procedure myocardial contrast echocardiography (MCE)
	Reasonable: Vigorous septal milking (consider cutting balloon technique)
	Contraindicated: Concomitant multivessel coronary disease that independently meets indications for coronary artery bypass grafting (CABG)
(Note: Patient must meet clinical, echocardiographic, *and* angiographic criteria.)	
NYHA, New York Heart Association; CCS, Canadian Cardiovascular Society.	

Echocardiographic criteria include basal septal wall hypertrophy of greater than 16–18 mm at the coaptation point of systolic anterior motion (SAM) of the mitral valve, asymmetric septal hypertrophy (ASH) (ratio of septum-to-posterior wall thickness >1.3:1), and concomitant SAM-related MR that is uniformly posteriorly directed (Fig. 12b.1).[8] The presence of central, anteriorly directed, or multiple-jet MR should prompt evaluation for an alternate etiology.[8] In most cases of significant MR, a transesophageal echocardiogram is required to confirm MR as SAM-related (Fig. 12b.2). A resting gradient of greater than 30 mm Hg and/or a provocable gradient more than 50–60 mm Hg must be documented.[1] Ideal candidates have focal basal hypertrophy or a "septal bulge" easily amenable to targeted alcohol infusion, leaving behind no additional areas for potential obstruction. Relative contraindications include severe septal thickening of greater than 30 mm and diffuse thickening extending into the mid-cavity (mid-cavity obstruction). Echocardiography should also evaluate for anomalous papillary muscles, redundant chords, subvalvular or supravalvular membranes, and abnormal papillary or chordal attachments (particularly to the basal septum) that would necessitate open surgical repair.[1,8]

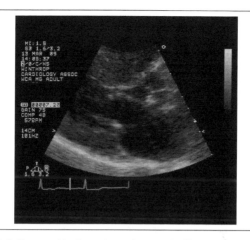

Figure 12b.1 Hypertrophic obstructive cardiomyopathy. Transthoracic echocardiographic parasternal long axis view shows asymmetric septal hypertrophy (ASH), systolic anterior motion of the anterior mitral valve leaflet (SAM), and likely resultant posteriorly directed mitral regurgitation (*not shown*).

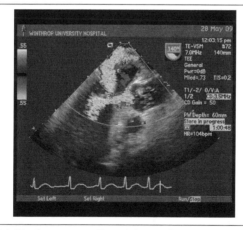

Figure 12b.2 Mitral regurgitation. Transesophageal echocardiography is necessary in patients with moderate to severe mitral regurgitation, in order to assess etiology of mitral regurgitation (MR). Mitral regurgitation due to hypertrophic obstructive cardiomyopathy and systolic anterior motion of the mitral valve results in posteriorly directed MR. Turbulence to flow in the outflow tract that divides into two separate jets (one into the aorta and the other posteriorly directed into the left atrium) results in the classic "Y" sign, indicating that MR is solely related to hypertrophic obstructive cardiomyopathy and is likely to respond to septal reduction therapy.

A thorough right and left heart catheterization while the patient is on optimal medical therapy should be performed. Alternative etiologies for the symptoms should be assessed, including pulmonary hypertension, severe volume overload, valvular disease, intracardiac shunts, and coronary disease. If a surgical indication is found, concomitant surgical myectomy should be the preferred treatment modality. Dynamic resting and provocable gradients are confirmed, the latter by premature ventricular contraction (Brockenbrough maneuver, Fig. 12b.3), Valsalva maneuver, or combination of the two.[9] Coronary angiography should pay particular attention to the presence or absence of septal perforators that enter the basal interventricular septum. The number, caliber, and length of septal perforators should be recorded (Fig. 12b.4). Perforators of at least 1.5 mm diameter are required for ethanol septal ablation.

Technique

Table 12b.2 lists the equipment necessary for successful ethanol septal ablation. Two transducers are required for simultaneous left ventricular (LV) and aorta pressure. It is important to document the highest resting and provocable gradient prior to the ablation, as success is determined by a greater than 50% reduction in gradient.[8,10] A 5 Fr temporary pacemaker is next advanced into the right ventricular (RV) apex and set for backup pacing. It is imperative that the pacer reach the RV apex, away from any potential infusion of alcohol. A guide catheter is chosen based on prior left heart catheterization, and advanced to the left main. Care must be taken to choose a guide with sufficient backup (e.g., XB or EBU), as the alcohol ablation procedure is performed through an inflated balloon without a wire in place.

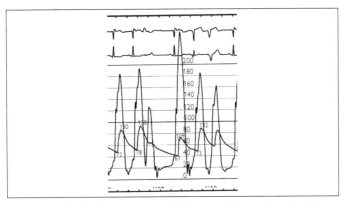

Figure 12b.3 **Brockenbrough maneuver.** Simultaneous left ventricular and aortic pressure tracings evidence a dynamic gradient. After a premature ventricular contraction, the subsequent tracing shows a rise in gradient and fall in pulse pressure, the classic Brockenbrough maneuver. A resting gradient of approximately 90 mm Hg rises to >200 mm Hg on provocation.

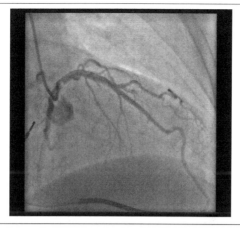

Figure 12b.4 Left coronary angiography. Right anterior oblique (RAO) cranial projection of left coronary angiography reveals the left anterior descending artery with multiple septal perforators. Two large septal perforators are shown and are possible candidates for ethanol septal ablation.

Table 12b.2 Required equipment for ethanol septal ablation
1. Two-transducer set-up to measure outflow tract gradient
2. Right heart catheter (Swan–Ganz)
3. Transvenous pacemaker
4. Left coronary guide catheter with appropriate back-up (6 Fr standard)
5. Pigtail catheter (5 Fr)
6. Long workhorse wire (operator's preference)
7. Anticoagulation (unfractionated heparin or bivalirudin)
8. Sedation and/or analgesia (i.e., morphine or versed)
9. Short (6–10 mm) over-the-wire balloon, 25% greater diameter than septal perforator
10. Echocardiographic or angiographic contrast
11. Two 5 cc vials of 98% ethanol (desiccated)
12. Standard arterial and venous femoral sheaths
13. Standard angioplasty equipment (i.e., Indeflator, insertion tool)
14. Transthoracic (standard) or intracardiac (advanced) echocardiography
15. Closure device (optional, i.e., Angio-Seal)
16. Over-the-wire cutting balloon in small diameter (2–2.5 × 6 mm) (optional)

The patient is anticoagulated with heparin (activated clotting time [ACT] > 250) or bivalirudin. Using a long workhorse wire (e.g., Asahi Soft or BMW), the presumed optimal septal perforator is wired and the wire tip placed as distally as possible. The stiff part of the wire must be at least 1 cm past the origin of the septal perforator to allow proper balloon positioning. A short (6–9 mm length) over-the-wire balloon approximately 25% larger in caliber than the perforator is placed in the proximal segment 1 mm past the ostium (Fig. 12b.5). An echocardiographic technician must be in position to check both parasternal and apical views of the basal septum. Since balloon inflation produces angina, morphine and/or versed should be available. The balloon is inflated to low atmosphere (typically 4–6 atm), the wire removed, and contrast injected through the central lumen. On echocardiography, the basal septum at the point of mitral valve contact should become echogenic, indicating appropriate opacification of the target myocardium. Fluoroscopy must document antegrade flow down the septal artery, lack of reflux into the left anterior descending (LAD) artery, and lack of distal flow into other territories, particularly the right posterior descending artery (PDA). If fluoroscopy shows reflux or distant vessel flow, or the echocardiogram fails to reveal opacification of target myocardium (or reveals opacification of distant sites such as the RV free wall, moderator band, or papillary muscle), then ablation is aborted. An adjacent septal perforator, if available, may be attempted. Figure 12b.6 shows acceptable myocardial contrast echocardiography (MCE).

If the perforator serves the appropriate area by MCE, 1–3 cc of ethanol is infused at a rate of 1 cc/min. Electrocardiogram (EKG) changes consistent with anterior ischemia may be noted, and the patient may develop chest pain. Morphine and/or versed may be given. During ethanol infusion, LAD angiography must document continued normal antegrade flow. Diminished flow indicates reflux of alcohol and mandates aborting the procedure. In addition, the patient may develop complete heart block. After ethanol, 0.5 cc of saline is infused through the lumen to clear the catheter of residual ethanol, the balloon is left inflated for an additional 5 minutes, and then removed.

Valsalva and/or Brockenbrough maneuvers should be repeated to document post-procedure resting and provoked gradients. If a 50% reduction in both resting and provoked gradients is obtained, or residual gradient is less than 30 mm Hg, the procedure is deemed successful.[8] Such reductions, especially if the residual gradient is less than 30 mm Hg, result in continued gradient reduction due to LV remodeling. If 50% reduction is not obtained, a second septal perforator may be interrogated and ablation performed if acceptable.[11]

Procedural Complications and In-hospital Care

Current procedural complications (exclusive of the need for permanent pacemaker) occur in fewer than 2% of patients, with mortality at 1.5%.[12] The main electrical finding is right bundle branch block, seen in 70%.[13] This is not surprising, as the right bundle is supplied by the LAD in over 90% of patients, and alcohol septal ablation typically infarcts the RV side of the interventricular septum.[14] Complete heart block requiring permanent pacemaker occurs in 5%–10%.[12] Risk factors include preexisting left bundle branch block, female gender, bolus injection of ethanol, large amount of ethanol, and injection of more than one perforator.[15] Transient complete heart block during the procedure is also predictive.[16] Complete heart block typically occurs within 12 hours, with the majority occurring within 3–4 days. In rare cases, complete heart block may

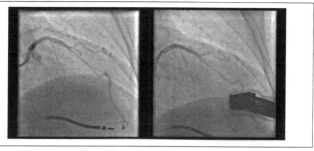

Figure 12b.5 Ethanol septal ablation. A wire is placed in the first septal perforator, with the opaque section as distal as possible. An appropriately sized balloon is positioned >1 mm past the septal perforator ostium and inflated. The wire will be removed and contrast injected for echo guidance, followed by ethanol infusion if the target myocardium is confirmed. On the right, an echo probe is seen on the chest wall.

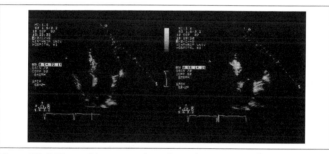

Figure 12b.6 Myocardial contrast echocardiographic guidance. Apical views before and after contrast infusion through the balloon central lumen, showing opacification limited to the basal septum at the point of outflow tract obstruction.

occur late, once the patient has been discharged. Predicting late heart block is the subject of active research.[16]

To monitor for complete heart block and ventricular arrhythmia, patients are maintained in the cardiac care unit for 48 hours. Cardiac enzymes should be monitored every 8 hours until peak (typical CK 800–1,800) and echocardiogram performed to document hypokinesis of the basal septum and immediate postprocedure result. During the initial 24 hours, the temporary pacemaker is left in place. In patients who already have a permanent implant (implantable cardioverter defibrillator [ICD] or pacemaker), this should be sufficient as long as the lead is not in the basal septum (area of ablation). If there is doubt, the output of the device may be increased as a precaution. All preprocedure medications should be restarted, including high-dose β-blocker or calcium channel blocker therapy.

If the patient develops complete heart block, a permanent pacemaker is implanted as early as possible, so that the patient may ambulate and be discharged on day 4. If no heart block develops, the temporary pacer is removed at 24 hours, the patient leaves the intensive care unit at 48 hours, and is similarly discharged on day 4.

Immediate, Intermediate, and Long-term Outcome

The comparative effectiveness of alcohol septal ablation and surgical myectomy is hotly debated, with no randomized controlled trials available; however, there is growing evidence that the procedure is successful in over 90% of appropriately selected patients.[1,6] Importantly, the development of complete heart block and requirement for pacemaker implantation does not impact success.[15] Figure 12b.7 shows the immediate gradient reduction obtained in the patient from Figure 12b.3. Typically, a triphasic response at the target myocardium has been noted, with initial infarction and stunning of the basal septum resulting in oftentimes complete resolution of gradient, followed by partial recurrence of gradient over the first week post-procedure as stunned myocardium begins to contract once more, and ultimately continued reduction of gradient once more as the infarcted myocardium thins and outflow tract widens. Figure 12b.8 shows the basal septum at 1–2 months postprocedure.

Intermediate and long-term outcomes are favorable, with improved functional status, quality of life, treadmill time, and reductions in septal thickness, outflow tract gradients, and MR out to 5 years.[17] Importantly, the abolition of outflow tract gradient and MR results in a regression of LV hypertrophy throughout the ventricle (not solely limited to the infarcted septum), a remodeling process that improves both diastolic function and clinical symptoms.[18] One concern with alcohol septal ablation has been the possibility of a late increase in mortality due to scar formation in the interventricular septum. However, case reports of sudden death after alcohol septal ablation have been rare. In addition, at least two studies of serial evoked potential testing before and after ablation have failed to indicate increased predilection for ventricular arrhythmia.[10,19] Further, rates of appropriate ICD discharge after ethanol septal ablation are lower than expected.[20,21]

Special Considerations

Ethanol septal ablation has been performed in patients with mid-cavitary obstruction and severe septal wall hypertrophy (>30 mm thickness). However, both have shown unpredictable success; the former due to the absolute mass of muscle that would need to be ablated to eliminate obstruction and the latter due to the difficulty inherent to matching the mid-cavitary septal muscle with available septal perforators. In addition, patients with extremely high gradients (>100 mm Hg resting gradient) have an unpredictable response.

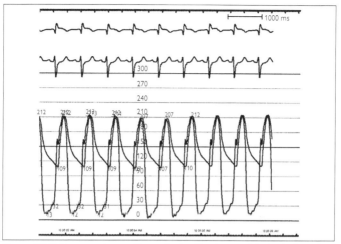

Figure 12b.7 Postprocedure gradient reduction. Simultaneous left ventricular and aortic pressure tracings post procedure reveal minimal residual resting gradient, without augmentation on Valsalva maneuver (second half of tracing). Note that this is the same patient whose preprocedure gradients are shown in Figure 12b.3.

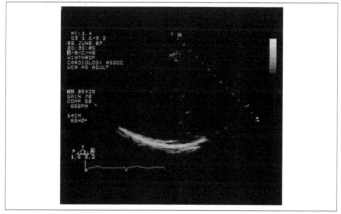

Figure 12b.8 Echocardiogram post procedure. Parasternal long axis view of a patient 1–2 months post ablation shows scar contraction of the basal septum and resultant widening of the left ventricular outflow tract. Obstruction and mitral regurgitation are no longer present (not shown).

In some cases, vigorous myocardial contractility results in septal "milking" of the perforators, with potentially catastrophic results if the balloon "watermelon-on-seeds" back into the LAD. Use of an over-the-wire short cutting balloon (2.0 × 6 mm or 2.5 × 6 mm) at low atmospheres fixes the balloon in the septal artery and facilitates a successful procedure.[22]

Surgical myectomy and ethanol septal ablation have been performed in the same patient, with reports of successful ablation after unsuccessful myectomy and successful myectomy after unsuccessful ablation.[11,23,24] The main complication, along with increased morbidity, is an increase in the need for a permanent pacemaker.[11]

In patients whose angiography fails to reveal optimal septal perforators arising from the LAD, a careful search for anomalous septal arteries should be performed. These may arise from a parallel running diagonal artery, the left main, or the proximal right coronary artery, and have facilitated successful ethanol septal ablation in experienced hands.[25]

Conclusion

Ethanol septal ablation is an accepted alternative to surgical myectomy in patients who meet strict clinical, echocardiographic, and angiographic criteria, with similar short- and intermediate-term outcomes. Recent literature continues to confirm the benefit of this procedure in improving outflow tract gradient, MR, and associated symptoms of dyspnea, angina, and presyncope/syncope, when performed by experienced operators.

Practical Pearls

- Always have extra vials of ethanol on hand in case multiple ablations are required.
- A transvenous pacemaker is always required, and it should be placed on the table even in cases with permanent implants.
- Guide backup is crucial, as inadvertent movement and slippage of the balloon will cause anterior myocardial infarction not amenable to treatment.
- Consider the cutting balloon in cases of vigorous septal contractility, in order to avoid balloon slippage back into the LAD during infusion.
- Stick to the 1 cc/min infusion rate. Slower infusions may lead to early coagulation of the artery without adequate ablation, whereas rapid infusions increase the risk of complete heart block.
- A small dose of intracoronary nitroglycerin (100 μg) infused through the guide may dilate septal perforators and aid in balloon sizing.
- When a transvenous pacemaker is left in place, using an arterial closure device may avoid inadvertent disengagement of the pacemaker.
- Continue all preprocedure medications, including high-dose β-blockers and calcium channel blockers, regardless of postprocedure conduction disease.
- Monday is the best day to perform alcohol ablations, as patients typically remain in the hospital 4 days, and this allows for timely placement of permanent pacemakers and increased ability to respond to complications.

References

1. Maron BJ, McKenna WJ, Danielson GK, et al. American College of Cardiology/European Society of Cardiology clinical expert consensus document on hypertrophic cardiomyopathy. *J Am Coll Cardiol.* 2003;42(9):1687-1713.

2. Maron BJ, Olivotto I, Spirito P, et al. Epidemiology of hypertrophic cardiomyopathy-related death: revisited in a large non-referral-based patient population. *Circulation.* 2000;102:858-864.

3. Maron MS, Olivotto I, Betocchi S, et al. Effect of left ventricular outflow tract obstruction on clinical outcome in hypertrophic cardiomyopathy. *N Engl J Med.* 2003;348:295-303.

4. Brown ML, Schaff HV. Surgical management of obstructive hypertrophic cardiomyopathy: the gold standard. *Expert Rev Cardiovasc Ther.* 2008;6(5):715-722.

5. Sigwart U. Non-surgical myocardial reduction for hypertrophic obstructive cardiomyopathy. *Lancet.* 1995;346:211-214.

6. Alam M, Dokainish H, Lakkis NM. Hypertrophic obstructive cardiomyopathy: alcohol septal ablation vs. myectomy: A meta-analysis. *Eur Heart J.* 2009;30(9):1080-1087.

7. Braunwald E, Seidman CE, Sigwart U. Contemporary evaluation and management of hypertrophic cardiomyopathy. *Circulation.* 2002;106:1312-1316.

8. Holmes DR Jr., Valeti US, Nishimura RA. Alcohol septal ablation for hypertrophic cardiomyopathy: indications and technique. *Catheter Cardiovasc Interv.* 2005;66:375-389.

9. Brockenbrough EC, Braunwald E, Morrow AG. A hemodynamic technic for the detection of hypertrophic subaortic stenosis. *Circulation.* 1961;23:189-194.

10. Gietzen FH, Leuner CJ, Raute-Kreinsen U, et al. Acute and long-term results after transcoronary ablation of septal hypertrophy (TASH): catheter interventional treatment for hypertrophic obstructive cardiomyopathy. *Eur Heart J.* 1999;20:1342-1354.

11. Nagueh SF, Buergler JM, Quinones MA, et al. Outcome of surgical myectomy after unsuccessful alcohol septal ablation for the treatment of patients with hypertrophic obstructive cardiomyopathy. *J Am Coll Cardiol.* 2007;50(8): 795-798.

12. Alam M, Dokainish H, Lakkis N. Alcohol septal ablation for hypertrophic obstructive cardiomyopathy: a systematic review of published studies. *J Interv Cardiol.* 2006;19(4):319-327.

13. Runquist LH, Nielson CD, Killip D, et al. Electrocardiographic findings after alcohol septal ablation therapy for obstructive hypertrophic cardiomyopathy. *Am J Cardiol.* 2002;90(9):1020-1022.

14. Talreja DR, Nishimura RA, Edwards WD, et al. Alcohol septal ablation vs. surgical septal myectomy: comparison of effects on atrioventricular conduction tissue. *J Am Coll Cardiol.* 2004;44(12):2329-2332.

15. Chang SM, Nagueh SF, Spencer WH 3rd, et al. Complete heart block: determinants and clinical impact in patients with hypertrophic obstructive cardiomyopathy undergoing nonsurgical septal reduction therapy. *J Am Coll Cardiol.* 2003;42(2):296-300.

16. Lawrenz T, Lieder F, Bartelsmeier M, et al. Predictors of complete heart block after transcoronary ablation of septal hypertrophy: results of a prospective electrophysiologic investigation in 172 patients with hypertrophic obstructive cardiomyopathy. *J Am Coll Cardiol.* 2007;49(24):2356-2363.

17. Fernandes VL, Nagueh SF, Wang W, et al. A prospective follow-up of alcohol septal ablation for symptomatic hypertrophic obstructive cardiomyopathy – The Baylor experience (1996–2002). *Clin Cardiol.* 2005;28(3):124-130.

18. van Dockum WG, Beek AM, ten Cate FJ, et al. Early onset and progression of left ventricular remodeling after alcohol septal ablation in hypertrophic obstructive cardiomyopathy. *Circulation.* 2005;111(19):2503-2508.

19. Boekstegers P, Steinbigler P, Molnar A, et al. Pressure-guided nonsurgical myocardial reduction induced by small septal infarctions in hypertrophic obstructive cardiomyopathy. *J Am Coll Cardiol.* 2001;38:846-853.

20. Cuoco FA, Spencer WH 3rd, Fernandes VL, et al. Implantable cardioverter-defibrillator therapy for primary prevention of sudden death after alcohol septal ablation of hypertrophic cardiomyopathy. *J Am Coll Cardiol.* 2008;52(21):1718-1723.

21. Noseworthy PA, Rosenberg MA, Fifer MA, et al. Ventricular arrhythmia following alcohol septal ablation for obstructive hypertrophic cardiomyopathy. *Am J Cardiol.* 2009;104(1):128-132.

22. Polin N, Feldman D, Naidu SS. Alcohol septal ablation for hypertrophic obstructive cardiomyopathy: novel application of the cutting balloon. *J Invasive Cardiol.* 2006;18(9):436-437.

23. Juliano N, Wong SC, Naidu SS. Alcohol septal ablation for failed surgical myectomy. *J Invasive Cardiol.* 2005;17(10):569-571.

24. Joyal D, Arab D, Chen-Johnston C, et al. Alcohol septal ablation after failed surgical myectomy. *Catheter Cardiovasc Interv.* 2007;69(7):999-1002.

25. Choi D, Dardano J, Naidu SS. Alcohol septal ablation through an anomalous right coronary septal perforator: first report and discussion. *J Invasive Cardiol.* 2009;21(6):106-109.

Chapter 12c

Percutaneous Valve Replacement

Inder M. Singh and Mehdi H. Shishehbor

Over 50,000 individuals undergo surgical aortic valve replacement (AVR) in the United States every year.[1,2] The average perioperative mortality for isolated AVR is 8.8% in patients over the age of 65 years.[1,2] Although AVR remains the current standard of care for treating severe aortic stenosis (AS), at least a third of eligible patients are deemed inoperable secondary to associated comorbidities and are relegated to a suboptimal strategy of medical management only.[1,3] Transcatheter aortic valve implantation (TAVI) is well suited to bridge this treatment gap and potentially even match the outcomes of surgical AVR with new device and technical iterations.[4] The role of TAVI in severe symptomatic AS is being tested in the pivotal Placement of AoRTic TraNscathetER Valve' (PARTNER) trial involving the Edwards SAPIEN valve (Fig. 12c.112c.1).[4,5] Similarly, the CoreValve ReValving system is awaiting U.S. Food and Drug Administration approval to start its pivotal trial in the United States.[6] Both the SAPIAN valve and CoreValve are being used extensively in Europe since they received the European Compliance (CE) mark approval in 2007, and it is estimated that 5,000 TAVIs have been performed to date.[6,7] In this chapter, we discuss contemporary techniques for TAVI.

Patient Management

Approach to the Patient

Because of its complex nature, TAVI requires close collaboration among the interventional cardiologist, imaging cardiologist, and cardiac and vascular surgeons. Echocardiographic data should be carefully reviewed for valve anatomy, hemodynamics, and coexisting lesions. Screening for iliofemoral vessel size, peripheral vascular disease, aortic calcification, and tortuosity by computed tomography (CT), magnetic resonance angiography, or digital angiography is critical. Patients who are considered for TAVI must meet certain clinical and technical criteria (Fig. 12c.1).[5]

A.

PARTNER TRIAL Trial

	Cohort A – high surgical risk		Cohort B – inoperable/extreme surgical risk	
	Surgical AVR	PAVR	PAVR	Medical ± BAV

	Inclusion criteria	Primary end points	Secondary end points
Cohort A	1) Predicted operative mortality ≥15% or STS score ≥10 2) Degenerative AS, MPG > 40 mm Hg, AVA <0.8 cm², jet velocity > 4 m/s 3) ≥NYHA II	Freedom from death at 1 y	Functional improvement Freedom from MACCE Valve dysfunction Length of index hospital stay Total hospital days at 1 y QOL Improved valve function
Cohort B	1) Risk of procedural death/serious, irreversible morbidity > 50% 2) No. 2 + 3 from above	Freedom from death during study duration	Functional improvement Freedom from MACCE Total hospital days at 1 y QOL Improved valve function

3. Exclusion criterial of the PARTNER trial

Uni-/bicuspid aortic valve	Active peptic ulcer or GI bleeding within 3 m
Myocardial infarction ≤1 m	Allergy to aspirin, ticlopidine, clopidogrel, or heparin
Mixed aortic valve diseases (AR≥3+)	Native aortic annulus <16 or >24 mm
Invasive cardiac procedure (<30 d (≤6 m if DES implanted)	Patient refused surgery
Preexisting prosthetic valve	CVA or TIA within 6 m
Mitral regurgitation ≥3+	Renal insufficiency or end-stage renal disease requiring dialysis
Blood dyscrasias	Life expectancy <12 m due to noncardiac comorbidities
Coronary artery disease requiring revascularization	Significant aortic disease (aneurysm, tortuosity, excessive atheroma, or stenosis) (applicable to transfemoral route only)
Hemodynamic instability requiring inotropics or mechanical assistance	Iliofemoral vessels <7 mm (transfemoral route only)
Need for any emergency surgery	Participating in another trial
Hypertrophic cardiomyopathy with or without obstruction	
Severe LV dysfunction (<20%)	
Intracardiac mass, thrombus, or vegetation	

MPG, Mean pressure gradient; AVA, aortic value area; NYHA, New York Heart Association; GI, gastrointestinal; AR, aortic regurgitation; DES, drug-eluting stent; CVA, erebrovascular accident; TIA, transient ischemic attack.

Figure 12c.1 Placement of aortic transcatheter valve (PARTNER); cohorts and inclusion/exclusion criteria. Reprinted from Chiam PT, Ruiz CE. Percutaneous transcatheter aortic valve implantation: evolution of the technology. *Am Heart J,* 2009;157(2):229-242, with permission of the publisher (Mosby/Elsevier).

Table 12c.1 Transcatheter-based aortic valve prostheses in clinical use

Transcatheter Aortic Valve	Company	Mechanism	Valve Type	Structure	Approach	Status
CoreValve ReValving System	CoreValve	Self-expanding	Bovine pericardial	Nitinol	Retrograde	CE mark in EU IDE pending in US
Cribier-Edwards	Edwards Lifesciences	Balloon expandable	Equine pericardial	Stainless steel	Antegrade Retrograde, Transapical	Was in clinical use but phased out
Edwards SAPIEN	Edwards Lifesciences	Balloon expandable	Bovine pericardial	Stainless steel	Retrograde Transapical	Phase III in US CE mark in EU
SAPIEN XT	Edwards Lifesciences	Balloon expandable	Bovine pericardial	Cobalt-chromium	Retrograde	Clinically used OUS

EU, European Union; IDE, Investigational Device Exemption; US, United States; OUS, Outside United States.

From Singh IM, Shishehbor MH, Christofferson RD, Tuzcu EM, Kapadia SR. Percutaneous treatment of aortic valve stenosis. *Cleve Clin J Med.* 2008;75(11):805-812. Reprinted with permission, Cleveland Clinic Center for Medical Art & Photography © 2008-2009. All rights reserved.

Devices

Several valves are now in various stages of human trials for TAVI (Tables 12c.1–12c.3). Of these, the Edwards valve series and CoreValve are most advanced in their clinical usage and have already accumulated a fair amount of short- and mid-term data, mainly from European centers, to support their use (Table 12c.4). Thus, these prostheses will be focus of this chapter, although a number of other percutaneous valves are currently in various stages of development.

Edwards Valves

The Edwards series began with the Cribier-Edwards prosthesis; it was the first TAVI in a human subject in 2002, but it is no longer being used.[8] This was followed by the SAPIEN prosthesis (Fig. 12c.2), which received the European compliance (CE) mark approval in September 2007.[4] This is a balloon-expandable stented prosthesis with a tri-leaflet bovine pericardial tissue valve sutured within a stainless steel tubular frame and lengthened fabric sealing cuff. It is available in two sizes: 23 mm and 26 mm for annulus sizes ranging from 18 to 24 mm. This valve is currently being evaluated in the PARTNER trial. The most recent iteration of the Edwards series is the balloon-expandable SAPIEN XT (Fig. 12c.2).[9] It has a cobalt-chromium frame with thinner struts and a sutured tri-leaflet bovine pericardium valve.[9] These features make the SAPIEN XT achieve greater radial strength and structural integrity, along with a more open design for a lower profile. The leaflets are scalloped and closed at rest to enhance valve durability.

CoreValve

The CoreValve series is a self-expanding 50-mm-long nitinol stent composed of three bovine pericardial leaflets mounted and sutured within the frame (Fig. 12c.3). Being self-expandable, the CoreValve can conform to different aortic valve sizes and can anchor well in the aortic annulus. It requires the aortic valve annulus diameter to be between 20 and 27 mm, and the ascending aorta diameter, at the sinotubular junction, to be smaller than 45 mm.[10] Since the first human CoreValve implant in 2005, the valve has undergone three iterations.[10] The second and third prototypes improved on the original prosthesis by adopting a three-segment design—a straight bottom portion,

Table 12c.2 Transcatheter-based aortic valve prostheses in phase II trials

Transcatheter Aortic Valve	Company	Mechanism	Valve Type	Structure	Approach
Direct Flow	Direct Flow Medical	Inflatable rings	Bovine pericardial	Non-metallic	Retrograde
Lotus	Sadra Medical	Self-expanding	Bovine pericardial	Nitinol	Retrograde

Table 12c.3 Transcatheter-based aortic valve prostheses implanted in first-in-man series (phase I)

Transcatheter Aortic Valve	Company	Mechanism	Valve Type	Structure	Approach	Status
Aortx	Hansen Medical	Self-expanding	Pericardial tissue	Nitinol	–	Temporary implants during AVR
Enable	ATS (3F)	Self-expanding	Pericardial tissue	Nitinol	–	Temporary implants during AVR
JenaClip	JenaValve Technology	Self-expanding	Pericardial tissue	Nitinol	–	Temporary implants during AVR
Paniagua	Endoluminal Technology Research	Balloon expandable and self-expanding	Pericardial tissue	Nitinol and stainless steel	Retrograde	First-in-man (permanent implant)
Perceval	Sorin Group	Self-expanding	Bovine pericardial	Nitinol	–	Temporary implants during AVR

AVR, surgical aortic valve replacement.

Table 12c.4 Selected published series of transcatheter aortic valve implantation

Transcatheter Aortic Valve	Valve Prosthesis (Approach)	No. of Patients Treated	Follow-up Duration in Months	Outcomes % (death[†]/ stroke/MI/ PPM)
Edwards transfemoral				
Cribier[18] (2004)	First-generation (TF antegrade)	6	2	66.7/NR/NR/ NR
Cribier[19] (2006)	First-generation (TF antegrade and retrograde)	36	6	37/0/0/NR
Webb[20] (2007)#	First- and second-generation	50	1	12/4/2/4
Webb[9] (2009)#	Second- and third-generation	25	1	0/8/0/0
Edwards transapical				
Svensson[21] (2008)	Second-generation	40	4.8	37.5/5/17.5/NR
Walther[22] (2008)	Second-generation	50	12	28.6/NR/NR/ NR
Ye[23] (2009)	Second-generation	26	12	34.6/4/4/12
Walther[24] (2009)ᶜ	Second-generation	25	12	28/0/NR/NR
Edwards combined*				
PARTNER EU[25] (2009)	Second-generation (TF retrograde and TA)	130	12	38/6.5/5/5.8
SOURCE[26] (2009)	Second-generation (TF retrograde and TA)	1038	1	8.5/2.5/0.5/7
Webb[27] (2009)	First-, second-, and third-generation (TF retrograde and TA)	168	12	26.2/4.2/NR/5.4
Himbert[28] (2009)	Second-generation (TF retrograde and TA)	75	12	22/?/?/?
CoreValve#				
Grube[10] (2008)	First-, second-, and third-generation	136	12	29.8/7.1/3.6/27.9
Piazza[29] (2008)	Third-generation	645	1	8/1.9/0.6/9.3

Table 12c.4 Continued

Transcatheter Aortic Valve	Valve Prosthesis (Approach)	No. of Patients Treated	Follow-up Duration in Months	Outcomes % (death[†]/ stroke/MI/ PPM)
Buellesfeld[30] (2009)	Third-generation	126	12	28.6/7.1/5.4/31.3
Direct Flow#				
Schofer[16] (2008)	First-generation	15	1	6.7/6.7/6.7/0

[†]Death represents all cause mortality.

#Only transfemoral retrograde approach used in these series.

^{ς}All patients in this series had previous open-heart surgery.

*Includes both transfemoral and transapical approaches.

^{ψ}Permanent pacemaker outcomes for 6 months only.

MI, myocardial infarction; PPM, permanent pacemaker; NR, not reported; TF, transfemoral; TA, transapical.

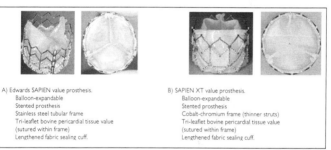

A) Edwards SAPIEN value prosthesis.
  Balloon-expandable
  Stented prosthesis
  Stainless steel tubular frame
  Tri-leaflet bovine pericardial tissue value
  (sutured within frame)
  Lengthened fabric sealing cuff.

B) SAPIEN XT value prosthesis.
  Balloon-expandable
  Stented prosthesis
  Cobalt-chromium frame (thinner struts)
  Tri-leaflet bovine pericardial tissue value
  (sutured within frame)
  Lengthened fabric sealing cuff.

Figure 12c.2 Edwards valve prostheses.

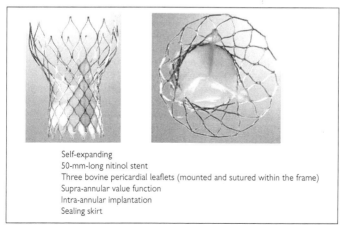

Self-expanding
50-mm-long nitinol stent
Three bovine pericardial leaflets (mounted and sutured within the frame)
Supra-annular value function
Intra-annular implantation
Sealing skirt

Figure 12c.3 CoreValve prosthesis.

which provides excellent radial force, excludes the calcified native leaflets, and avoids recoil; a tapered middle portion, which carries the valve itself and, by design, spares the coronary ostia; and a flared upper portion, which anchors the prosthesis in the ascending aorta and prevents it from migrating or embolizing. These iterations also significantly reduced the prosthesis profile. The latest prototype comes in a 26 mm size prosthesis for a 20–24 mm annulus and a 29 mm prosthesis for a 24–27 mm annulus. CoreValve may also offer limited repositioning capability since it is not a one-shot deployment. CoreValve received the European CE mark approval in May 2007.[4]

Detailing Techniques

General

The procedure can be performed via the femoral artery, vein, or by the transapical approach. However, the femoral artery (retrograde) approach is most widely used and is currently being performed with sedation and analgesia, whereas the transapical procedures are done under general anesthesia.[9,10] Heparin is used intraprocedurally and patients are premedicated with aspirin (81–325 mg) and clopidogrel (300–600 mg), which are continued indefinitely at standard maintenance doses (clopidogrel 75 mg/day).[9,10] Antibiotic prophylaxis is used.[9]

Access to Valve

Transvenous (femoral) antegrade, transarterial (femoral) retrograde, and transapical antegrade have all been used for TAVI. Of these, the antegrade approach, which was the approach in the first reported human TAVI in 2002,[8] has largely been abandoned due to technical challenges and potential mitral valve injury resulting in mitral regurgitation.[4] Currently, TAVI is performed through the transfemoral retrograde and transapical antegrade approaches.

Retrograde Technique

The retrograde technique starts with femoral artery access via a surgical cutdown or the standard Seldinger technique.[11] Sheath size is predetermined based on annular diameter, device type, and device size (18–24 Fr). In the past, surgical closure was the norm, but increasingly access site hemostasis is being obtained via preclosure devices to achieve a truly "percutaneous" procedure (Prostar XL, Abbott Vascular, Boston, MA). Serial dilations are followed by insertion of a long sheath that extends into the descending aorta and thus avoids device-related injury to the iliofemoral system.

Transapical Technique

The transapical technique is utilized in patients with severe vascular disease of the aorta or iliofemoral system.[12] A left anterolateral mini-thoracotomy is performed to expose the apex of the heart. Then two to three purse string sutures are placed in the LV apex, while taking care to avoid the coronaries. Access to the LV cavity is obtained via direct needle puncture followed by sheath insertion, through the purse string sutures, into the left ventricular (LV) cavity. Sheath size is predetermined as described earlier (21 or 26 Fr). After valve deployment, the sheath is removed and the purse string sutures are tied. This procedure should be performed in a hybrid operative suite. Potential disadvantages are LV and coronary injury, pericardial complications, and the need for general anesthesia plus chest tubes.

Preimplantation

The severely stenotic aortic valve is first prepared with traditional balloon aortic valvuloplasty using a Z-med II balloon catheter (NuMed Inc., Hopkinton, NY) that is sized 100%–110% of the annular diameter. This is performed over a Landerquest or Super Stiff Amplatz wire. Generally, the aortic valve is crossed using a 5 Fr AL-1 diagnostic catheter and a straight wire. Once in the LV, the straight wire is exchanged for the stiff wire, as noted earlier. The delivery system is then delivered.

Delivery System

The delivery system containing the valve prosthesis is advanced as a single unit to the level of the diseased aortic valve over a Lunderquist extra-stiff guidewire (Cook Medical, Bloomington, IN) or Super Stiff Amplatz (Boston Scientific, Watertown, MA). Each of these devices and techniques has a custom-made delivery system.

The RetroFlex 2 is a manually activated deflectable-tip delivery catheter currently used in the transfemoral retrograde approach for both SAPIEN and SAPIEN XT valves (Fig. 12c.4).[9] The aortic valve prosthesis is mounted over the 3-cm-long balloon catheter using a specially designed mechanical crimping device (NuMed Inc., Hopkinton, NY). Currently, an 18 Fr RetroFlex4 delivery system is in preclinical development.[9] The Ascendra delivery catheter is used in the transapical approach for both SAPIEN and SAPIEN XT.[12] It is currently available in a 26 Fr profile, and it is shorter in length compared to the transfemoral system.

The CoreValve Revalving retrograde delivery system consists of a loading/release handle, 12 Fr shaft, and an 18 Fr capsule that houses the CoreValve (Fig. 12c.5). This 18 Fr ReValving delivery system is currently employed for the arterial approach.[13] A 21 Fr system has recently been designed for the transapical approach, and the first-in-man procedure with that system was recently performed.[14]

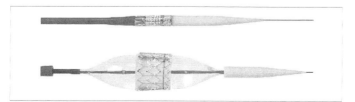

Figure 12c.4 RetroFlex2 delivery system for Edwards prostheses.

Implantation Technique

Prior to the implantation, anatomic landmarks are simultaneously evaluated by utilizing information from three imaging modalities: fluoroscopy for calcification of the native aortic valve leaflets and annulus; supravalvular aortogram for aortic cusps alignment plane and coronary ostia takeoff; and transesophageal echocardiography (TEE) for the LV outflow tract and mitral valve apparatus.

The Edwards valve prosthesis (SAPIEN or SAPIEN XT) contained in the Retroflex2 delivery system is advanced through the native valve such that the crimped valve lies at the level of the aortic annulus (Fig. 12c.6). The deflectable pusher portion is retracted into the ascending aorta, and the nose cone portion is advanced in the LV out flow tract. This exposes the deployment balloon and the overlying (crimped) prosthesis, which is positioned within the native

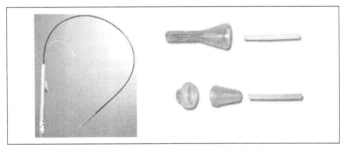

Figure 12c.5 Revalving delivery system for CoreValve prosthesis.

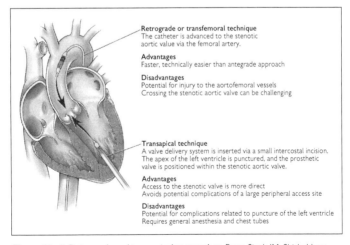

Retrograde or transfemoral technique
The catheter is advanced to the stenotic aortic valve via the femoral artery.

Advantages
Faster, technically easier than antegrade approach

Disadvantages
Potential for injury to the aortofemoral vessels
Crossing the stenotic aortic valve can be challenging

Transapical technique
A valve delivery system is inserted via a small intercostal incision. The apex of the left ventricle is punctured, and the prosthetic valve is positioned within the stenotic aortic valve.

Advantages
Access to the stenotic valve is more direct
Avoids potential complications of a large peripheral access site

Disadvantages
Potential for complications related to puncture of the left ventricle
Requires general anesthesia and chest tubes

Figure 12c.6 Retrograde and transapical approaches. From Singh IM, Shishehbor MH, Christofferson RD, Tuzcu EM, Kapadia SR. Percutaneous treatment of aortic valve stenosis. *Cleve Clin J Med.* 2008;75(11):805-812, with permission of the publisher (Cleveland Clinic Center for Medical Art & Photography).

valve using trimodal imaging, as described earlier. The optimal predeployment position for the Edwards valve is subannular, with two-thirds below the valve and one-third above the valve. The valve is then deployed under rapid right ventricular pacing (180–220 beats/min) to abruptly decrease transvalvular flow and facilitates precise deployment of the prosthesis (Figs. 12c.7 and 12c.8).

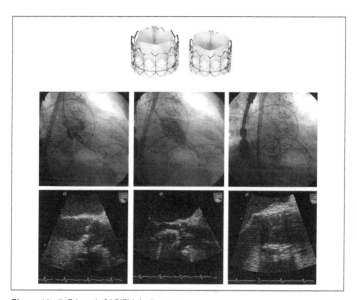

Figure 12c.7 Edwards SAPIEN deployment.

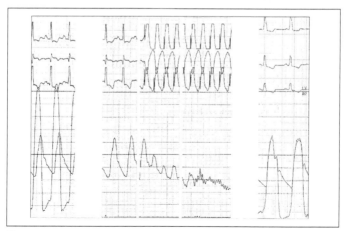

Figure 12c.8 Hemodynamic and pacing effects.

During deployment (Fig. 12c.7), the prosthesis typically moves forward and ideally rests at the mid-position of the aortic valve, which does not impinge the coronary ostia or impede the motion of the anterior mitral leaflet (Fig. 12c.9). The delivery system is then removed. The main difference between the final steps of the transapical versus transfemoral deployment is that, in the transapical approach, the valve is mounted in the antegrade direction on the shorter Ascendra delivery catheter (Fig. 12c.6). The rest of the steps are essentially the same.

The CoreValve delivery system is advanced across the predilated aortic valve. The valve is positioned such that only one or two cells of the prosthesis are under the annulus (Fig. 12c.10). The optimal position is one in which the prosthesis is intervalvular but the leaflets of the prosthesis sit just above the native leaflets in a supravalvular position (Fig. 12c.10). The origin of the coronary ostia is carefully avoided, and the flared top portion of the prosthesis anchors to the ascending aorta by design (Fig. 12c.10). Once optimal position is confirmed, using trimodal imaging, the prosthesis is unsheathed completely (Fig. 12c.11). No rapid right ventricular pacing is required for self-expanding prostheses.

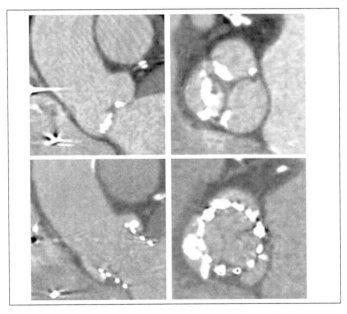

Figure 12c.9 Cardiac computed tomography, pre and post transcatheter aortic valve implantation.

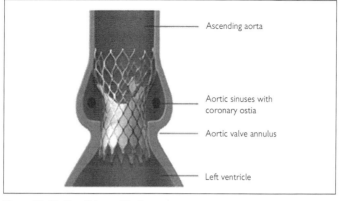

Figure 12c.10 CoreValve positioning

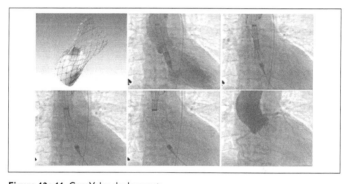

Figure 12c.11 CoreValve deployment.

Postimplant

After TAVI, aortography is necessary to assess the location and degree of aortic regurgitation, to confirm coronary patency, and to rule out complications such as hemopericardium or aortic dissection. Similarly, post-TAVI TEE is needed to evaluate the integrity of the LV out flow and mitral valve apparatus. Post-TAVI patients should be monitored closely in the cardiac intensive care unit for 24–48 hours, and then in a cardiac step-down unit for hemodynamic compromise, late conduction block, vascular complication, and renal failure. Patients continue taking aspirin indefinitely and clopidogrel for 3–6 months.

Special Issues

Procedure-related Complications

- Vascular complications continue to plague TAVI.[15] Rigorous screening with subsequent conversion to a transapical approach in cases of vascular abnormalities is a reasonable alternative until device and delivery systems have lower profiles.

- Stroke rates are still about 8% periprocedurally in the transfemoral retrograde approach.[15] Special attention to sheath and anticoagulation may help minimize these. Aortic arch filters are in development to prevent cerebral showering of aortic debris.

Device-related Complications

- Paravalvular leaks are more common, in both number and degree, in the Edwards SAPIEN valve.[15] However, the newer percutaneous valves, such as Direct Flow and Lotus, are significantly decreasing this problem.[16,17]

- Atrioventricular conduction blocks and need for a permanent pacemaker seem to be more common with CoreValve prosthesis.[15] This may be due to the prosthesis impinging on the interventricular septum, which contains the conduction system. Shorter second-generation devices may be able to address this issue.[16,17]

- Device embolization is much less of an issue as operator experience with optimal deployment and device stabilization has increased.[15] Also, newer devices have significantly higher radial force by design, making them more stably seated in the annulus.[16,17]

Conclusion

Severe symptomatic AS is a relatively common problem, with an increasing incidence as the population ages.[1,2] Surgical AVR provides excellent results, but it may have up to 13% mortality in the elderly population.[1] About 33% of individuals eligible for AVR are deemed inoperable due to significant comorbidities. Transcatheter aortic valve implantation may bridge the treatment gap in many of these patients. However, as with any procedure, appropriate patient selection and screening is paramount to achieving meaningful short- and long-term outcomes with TAVI.[3–5,14,15]

Given patient and procedural complexities, a collaborative effort among interventionalists, cardiac and vascular surgeons, and imaging specialists will be in the best interests of the patient. Multimodality imaging is a key to procedural success, preventing complications and recognizing them when they occur.[4,5,14,15]

The field is moving forward rapidly, and to date more than 5000 TAVIs have been performed.[7] Although this is an exciting time, with encouraging short- to mid-term outcomes, the risk of endocarditis, thromboembolic events, and the feasibility of subsequent aortic valve intervention are not known. Our enthusiasm should be tempered until the durability of the procedures and devices are established through multicenter randomized controlled trials.

Practical Pearls

- In general, the prostheses should be oversized relative to the annulus to minimize paravalvular regurgitation and prevent embolization.
- Postdilatation with a slightly larger balloon catheter may reduce paravalvular regurgitation.
- Sedation and analgesia are preferred for the transfemoral approach. This approach may prevent the adverse events related to general anesthesia.

References

1. Bonow RO, Carabello BA, Chatterjee K, et al. 2008 focused update incorporated into the ACC/AHA 2006 guidelines for the management of patients with valvular heart disease: a report of the American College of Cardiology/American Heart Association Task Force on Practice Guidelines (Writing Committee to revise the 1998 guidelines for the management of patients with valvular heart disease). Endorsed by the Society of Cardiovascular Anesthesiologists, Society for Cardiovascular Angiography and Interventions, and Society of Thoracic Surgeons. *J Am Coll Cardiol.* 2008;52(13):e1-142.

2. Nkomo VT, Gardin JM, Skelton TN, et al. Burden of valvular heart diseases: a population-based study. *Lancet.* 2006;368(9540):1005-1011.

3. Iung B, Baron G, Butchart EG, et al. A prospective survey of patients with valvular heart disease in Europe: The Euro Heart Survey on Valvular Heart Disease. *Eur Heart J.* 2003;24(13):1231-1243.

4. Singh IM, Shishehbor MH, Christofferson RD, Tuzcu EM, Kapadia SR. Percutaneous treatment of aortic valve stenosis. *Cleve Clin J Med.* 2008;75(11): 805-812.

5. Chiam PT, Ruiz CE. Percutaneous transcatheter aortic valve implantation: evolution of the technology. *Am Heart J.* 2009;157(2):229-242.

6. Shishehbor MH, Tuzcu EM, Kapadia SR. Percutaneous balloon valvuloplasty, valve replacement and valve repair. In: Lewis RP, ed. *Adult Clinical Cardiology Self-Assessment Program (ACCSAP) 7.* Bethesda, MD: American College of Cardiology Foundation, 2009.

7. Thomas M, Wendler O. Transcatheter aortic valve implantation (TAVI): how to interpret the data and what data is required? *EuroIntervention.* 2009;5(1):25-27.

8. Cribier A, Eltchaninoff H, Bash A, et al. Percutaneous transcatheter implantation of an aortic valve prosthesis for calcific aortic stenosis: first human case description. *Circulation.* 2002;106(24):3006-3008.

9. Webb JG, Altwegg L, Masson JB, et al. A new transcatheter aortic valve and percutaneous valve delivery system. *J Am Coll Cardiol.* 2009;53(20):1855-1858.

10. Grube E, Buellesfeld L, Mueller R, et al. Progress and current status of percutaneous aortic valve replacement: results of three device generations of the CoreValve revalving system. *Circ Cardiovasc Intervent.* 2008;1(3):167-175.

11. Webb JG, Chandavimol M, Thompson CR, et al. Percutaneous aortic valve implantation retrograde from the femoral artery. *Circulation*. 2006;113(6): 842-850.

12. Lichtenstein SV, Cheung A, Ye J, et al. Transapical transcatheter aortic valve implantation in humans: initial clinical experience. *Circulation*. 2006;114(6): 591-596.

13. Grube E, Laborde JC, Gerckens U, et al. Percutaneous implantation of the CoreValve self-expanding valve prosthesis in high-risk patients with aortic valve disease: the Siegburg first-in-man study. *Circulation*. 2006;114(15):1616-1624.

14. Vahanian A, Alfieri O, Al-Attar N, et al. Transcatheter valve implantation for patients with aortic stenosis: a position statement from the European Association of Cardio-Thoracic Surgery (EACTS) and the European Society of Cardiology (ESC), in collaboration with the European Association of Percutaneous Cardiovascular Interventions (EAPCI). *Eur Heart J*. 2008;29(11):1463-1470.

15. Zajarias A, Cribier AG. Outcomes and safety of percutaneous aortic valve replacement. *J Am Coll Cardiol*. 2009;53(20):1829-1836.

16. Schofer J, Schlüter M, Treede H, et al. Retrograde transarterial implantation of a nonmetallic aortic valve prosthesis in high-surgical-risk patients with severe aortic stenosis. a first-in-man feasibility and safety study. *Circ Cardiovasc Intervent*. 2008;1:126-133.

17. Buellesfeld L, Gerckens U, Grube E. Percutaneous implantation of the first repositionable aortic valve prosthesis in a patient with severe aortic stenosis. *Catheter Cardiovasc Interv*. 2008;71(5):579-584.

18. Cribier A, Eltchaninoff H, Tron C, et al. Early experience with percutaneous transcatheter implantation of heart valve prosthesis for the treatment of end-stage inoperable patients with calcific aortic stenosis. *J Am Coll Cardiol*. 2004;43(4):698-703.

19. Cribier A, Eltchaninoff H, Tron C, et al. Treatment of calcific aortic stenosis with the percutaneous heart valve: mid-term follow-up from the initial feasibility studies: the French experience. *J Am Coll Cardiol*. 2006;47(6):1214-1223.

20. Webb JG, Pasupati S, Humphries K, et al. Percutaneous transarterial aortic valve replacement in selected high-risk patients with aortic stenosis. *Circulation*. 2007;116(7):755-763.

21. Svensson LG, Dewey T, Kapadia S, et al. United States feasibility study of transcatheter insertion of a stented aortic valve by the left ventricular apex. *Ann Thorac Surg*. 2008;86(1):46-54; discussion 54-45.

22. Walther T, Falk V, Kempfert J, et al. Transapical minimally invasive aortic valve implantation; the initial 50 patients. *Eur J Cardiothorac Surg*. 2008;33(6):983-988.

23. Ye J, Cheung A, Lichtenstein SV, et al. Transapical transcatheter aortic valve implantation: 1-year outcome in 26 patients. *J Thorac Cardiovasc Surg*. 2009;137(1):167-173.

24. Walther T, Falk V, Borger MA, et al. Transapical aortic valve implantation in patients requiring redo surgery. *Eur J Cardiothorac Surg*. 2009;36(2):231-234; discussion 234-235.

25. Schachinger V, Lefevre T, De Bruyne B, et al. Results from the PARTNER EU trial: Primary endpoint analysis. *Presented at EuroPCR*. Barcelona, Spain, 2009.

26. Thomas M, Schymik G, Walther T, et al. 30 day results of the SOURCE registry: a European registry of transcatheter aortic valve implantation using the Edwards SAPIEN valve. *Presented at EuroPCR*. Barcelona, Spain, 2009.

27. Webb JG, Altwegg L, Boone RH, et al. Transcatheter aortic valve implantation: impact on clinical and valve-related outcomes. *Circulation.* 2009;119(23):3009-3016.

28. Himbert D, Descoutures F, Al-Attar N, et al. Results of transfemoral or transapical aortic valve implantation following a uniform assessment in high-risk patients with aortic stenosis. *J Am Coll Cardiol.* 2009;54(4):303-311.

29. Piazza N, Grube E, Gerckens U, et al. Procedural and 30-day outcomes following transcatheter aortic valve implantation using the third generation (18 Fr) CoreValve revalving system: results from the multicentre, expanded evaluation registry 1-year following CE mark approval. *EuroIntervention.* 2008;4(2):242-249.

30. Buellesfeld L. 12 months safety and performance results of transcatheter aortic valve implantation using the 18F CoreValve Revalving prosthesis. *Presented at EuroPCR.* Barcelona, Spain, 2009.

Index

265

Printed in the USA/Agawam, MA
November 15, 2012

570398.090